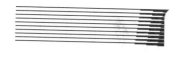

BLS Case Studies in Emergency Care

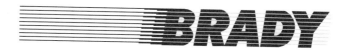

BLS Case Studies in Emergency Care

Daniel Limmer, EMT-P
Paramedic, Kennebunk Fire Rescue
Kennebunk, Maine
Adjunct Faculty, Southern Maine Community College
South Portland, Maine

with

Shawn Salter, RN, NREMT-P, FP-C
Chief Flight Nurse and Director of Clinical Operations
San Antonio AirLife
San Antonio, Texas

and

Stephen Rahm, NREMT-P
Kendall County EMS Training Institute
Boerne, Texas

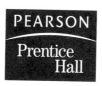

PEARSON
Prentice Hall

Upper Saddle River, New Jersey 07458

Library of Congress Cataloging-in-Publication Data

Limmer, Daniel.
    BLS case studies in emergency care / Daniel Limmer, with Shawn Salter and Stephen Rahm.
        p. ; cm.
    Includes index.
    ISBN 0-8359-5389-0 (alk. paper)
    1. Medical emergencies—Case studies.
    [DNLM: 1. Emergency Treatment—methods. 2. Case Reports. 3. Emergencies. WB 105
    L733b 2005] I. Salter, Shawn. II. Rahm, Stephen J. III. Title.
    RC86.7.L558 2005
    616.02'5—dc22

                                                    2004024734

Publisher: Julie Levin Alexander
Publisher's Assistant: Regina Bruno
Executive Editor: Marlene McHugh Pratt
Senior Managing Editor for Development: Lois Berlowitz
Project Manager: Andrea Edwards, Triple SSS Press
Editorial Assistant: Matthew Sirinides
Director of Marketing: Karen Allman
Senior Marketing Manager: Katrin Beacom
Channel Marketing Manager: Rachele Strober
Marketing Coordinator: Michael Sirinides
Director of Production and Manufacturing: Bruce Johnson

Managing Editor for Production: Patrick Walsh
Production Liaison: Faye Gemmellaro
Production Editor: Melissa Scott/Carlisle Publishers Services
Manufacturing Manager: Ilene Sanford
Manufacturing Buyer: Pat Brown
Creative Director: Cheryl Asherman
Senior Design Coordinator: Christopher Weigand
Cover Designer: Christopher Weigand
Printing and Binding: Courier Stoughton
Cover Printer: Phoenix Color

Notice: The author and the publisher of this book have taken care to make certain that the information given is correct and compatible with the standards generally accepted at the time of publication. Nevertheless, as new information becomes available, changes in treatment and in the use of equipment and procedures become necessary. The reader is advised to carefully consult the instruction and information material included in each piece of equipment or device before administration. Students are warned that the use of any techniques must be authorized by their medical advisor, where appropriate, in accordance with local laws and regulations. The publisher disclaims any liability, loss, injury, or damage incurred as a consequence, directly or indirectly, of the use and application of any of the contents of this book.

Studentaid.ed.gov, the U.S. Department of Education's website on college planning assistance, is a valuable tool for anyone intending to pursue higher education. Designed to help students at all stages of schooling, including international students, returning students, and parents, it is a guide to the financial aid process. The website presents information on applying to and attending college as well as on funding your education and repaying loans. It also provides links to useful resources, such as state education agency contact information, assistance in filling out financial aid forms, and an introduction to various forms of student aid.

Pearson Education Ltd.
Pearson Education Singapore, Pte. Ltd.
Pearson Education Canada, Ltd.
Pearson Education—Japan

Pearson Education Australia Pty., Limited
Pearson Education North Asia Ltd.
Pearson Educación de Mexico, S.A. de C.V.
Pearson Education Malaysia, Pte. Ltd.
Pearson Education Upper Saddle River, NJ

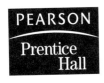

10 9 8 7 6 5 4 3 2 1
ISBN 0-8359-5389-0

CONTENTS

PREFACE

Initial education for the EMT often consists of frenzied learning of facts and skills in preparation for an examination that will determine whether you will obtain your license or certification. This provides you a significant amount of knowledge and an equally significant lack of street experience to apply what you have learned.

It would be quite convenient if patients always demonstrated the exact symptoms listed in your textbook (in the same order as the bullet points). Unfortunately, this is rarely the case. You are faced with the daunting task of linking your classroom and skill learning with the street. This is the main purpose of this book—to bring together classroom knowledge and street skills.

These case studies answer three questions that will be valuable to the new or experienced EMT: How, Why, and Application.

How—How real patients present on real calls. These cases are culled from the experience of EMS practitioners and educators to provide a realistic look at how you will find real patients and problems.

Why—Why do patients present as they do? Why does one condition mimic another? These cases will take you on a practical exploration of common and not-so-common calls. The Patient Outcome/Pathophysiology section at the end of each case offers an explanation of the events of the call, the patient outcome, and how the medical or traumatic condition affected the patient.

Application—You will apply your knowledge to real-life situations. You will be given information, observations, complaints, and physical assessment findings and be asked to make decisions based on this information—just as on a real call.

USING THIS TEXT

Each of the 44 cases presented in this book describes a real-life situation. You will begin each case with scene size-up and initial impression. This sets the foundation for a call. Are there dangers? Is the patient critical? You will decide.

During the assessment and care for the patient section of each case, you will be asked important questions. Try to consider these questions yourself without looking forward to the answer provided in the text. The material you have read plus the answer sets the foundation for the next portion of the scenario. You will transport and hand-off your patient to the emergency department staff.

There is more to EMS than hands-on patient care, and this book covers all of the angles. You will be exposed to medication errors, partner conflicts, and some curves thrown into what appear to be routine calls—much like what actually occurs in the street.

The need to take exams and apply information on your exams is not neglected. Each scenario ends with 10 multiple-choice questions to help you synthesize your knowledge and test what you have learned.

For additional resources, please visit www.bradybooks.com.

ACKNOWLEDGMENTS

Two experienced EMS professionals contributed a great number of the case studies to this book. In this effort, both you, the reader, and I benefit from the experience and talent of Shawn Salter and Steve Rahm. Shawn is Chief Flight Nurse with San Antonio Airlife in San Antonio, Texas, and Steve is with the Kendall County EMS Training Institute in Boerne, Texas. I am additionally grateful to our reviewers, who helped keep us on track, checking that the cases are accurate as well as interesting. Very special thanks go to Alyson Emery, with Kennebunk Fire Rescue, who reviewed the page proofs as a final check. She also listens to my frequent ramblings at Kennebunk Fire Rescue while she should be working. I appreciate that.

My family has been wonderful in accepting my travels and hours up in the office. My wife Stephanie and daughter Sarah are most precious in my life; what I do has no meaning without them. I received considerable moral support in my office from my two big, goofy dogs Theo and Ruthie.

I would also like to express appreciation to the people at Brady. This book was conceived many years ago, long before it ever saw ink and paper, with the help of Judy Streger. Most recently Marlene Pratt has offered support and guidance in bringing this project to completion. Andrea Edwards of Triple SSS Press Media Development collected the manuscript as it flowed in, and she massaged the case studies into the book you see before you now. The design and production departments at Brady also played an important role in helping to make this book a reality.

The world has become a different place since I started writing books. What we do today is different in many ways. The dangers we face and the potential threats are greater than ever. Yet, as EMS providers we go from call to call taking care of our patients on an individual basis. Many of our patients need more handholding than astute clinical decision-making. May we never forget how to care for patients as we stay safe and wait for the "big one." What we do is special. Where we do it—in the street, in homes, fields, factories and farms—is special. Never forget that.

This book is dedicated to you, the EMT who goes out there every day and takes care of people. That is what EMS is all about.

INSTRUCTOR REVIEWERS

The reviewers of this text have provided many excellent suggestions and ideas for improving the text. The quality of the reviews has been outstanding, and the reviews have been a major aid in the preparation of the manuscript. The assistance provided by these EMT experts is deeply appreciated.

Vicki Bacidore, RN, MS
Loyola Emergency Medical Services
Loyola University Medical Center
Maywood, Illinois

Heather Collins
Treasure Valley Community College
Ontario, Oregon

Robert Hawkes
Southern Maine Community College
South Portland, Maine

Stanley Johnson
Northern Virginia Community College
Alexandria, Virginia

Jeanine Riner, MHSA, BS, RRT, NREMT-P
EMS Instructor
Swainsboro Technical College
Swainsboro, Georgia

Paul Salway
Southern Maine Community College
South Portland, Maine

ABOUT THE AUTHOR

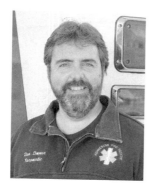

Dan Limmer, EMT-P, has been involved in EMS for over 25 years. He remains active as a paramedic with Kennebunk Fire Rescue in Kennebunk, Maine, and the Kennebunkport EMS (KEMS) in Kennebunkport, Maine. A passionate educator, Dan teaches EMT and paramedic courses at the Southern Maine Community College in South Portland, Maine, and has taught at The George Washington University in Washington, DC, and the Hudson Valley Community College in Troy, New York. He is a charter member of the National Association of EMS Educators and a member of the National Association of EMTs (NAEMT), for which he serves on the Advanced Medical Life Support Committee.

Dan was formerly involved in law enforcement, beginning as a dispatcher and retiring as a police officer in Colonie, New York, where he received three command recognition awards as well as the distinguished service award (Officer of the Year) in 1987. During his 20-year law enforcement career he served in the communications, patrol, juvenile, narcotics, and training units.

In addition to authoring several EMS journal articles, Dan is co-author of a number of EMS textbooks for Brady including *First Responder: A Skills Approach*, *Essentials of Emergency Care*, *Advanced Medical Life Support*, the military and fire service editions of *Emergency Care*, and others. He speaks frequently at regional, state, and national EMS conferences.

1

My Mother Is Gone

Objectives

At the conclusion of this scenario, the participant will be able to:

1. List four signs of obvious death.

2. Describe the involvement of medical control when dealing with an obvious death.

3. Define and apply procedures of the following in relation to the cardiac arrest patient:
   - "Do not resuscitate" orders
   - Pronouncing death

SCENARIO

You are summoned to 105 Mesquite Avenue at 1745 for a patient of unknown age who is "not breathing." Your response time to the scene is approximately 8 minutes.

1. When you are responding to such a call, what discussion(s) should you and your partner be having while en route?

   Preparation! You could be responding for anything from a witnessed cardiac arrest to an obviously deceased person and everything in between. Unfortunately, you have limited information at this point and do not know exactly what to take to the scene; therefore, prepare for the worst. At a minimum, you must bring your automated external defibrillator (AED) and adequate airway management equipment that must be able to manage patients ranging from the neonate to the elderly.

Having already donned your gloves, you arrive on the scene at 1754. You carry your equipment, including an AED, to the front door and are met by a middle-aged man who states, "My mother is gone." He begins to lead you to an upstairs bedroom.

2. As you are being lead to the bedroom, you are reviewing your priorities of initial assessment and management. What are they?

    First of all, you haven't even established that the patient is "gone," as the son has stated, so your routine initial assessment of the ABCs (Airway, Breathing and Circulation) will determine how you proceed with the management of the patient. At this point, you should be considering two things: first, the possibility that the patient is indeed in cardiac arrest and that your AED will be the most important initial piece of equipment; and second, you should consider the need for additional personnel (preferably advanced life support [ALS]) should this turn out to be a "workable" full cardiac arrest.

    You and your partner enter the room, where you see an emaciated elderly woman lying supine in a hospital bed. Her eyes are open and have a "glazed" appearance. The son states that his mother has been suffering from terminal brain cancer and that her physician gave her approximately 1 week to live. Her physician last saw her 4 days ago.

3. With this new information, has the priority of your management considerations changed?

    Not in terms of the initial assessment. Emergency medical technicians (EMTs) must perform an initial assessment on all patients they encounter. At this point, however, since the patient is suffering from an apparently terminal illness, you should be thinking of the possibility of an advanced directive such as a "do not resuscitate" order, also known as a DNR and, based upon the patient's history and the findings of your initial assessment, asking the son if one exists. In some systems, a DNR order must be "validated" by a physician, either in person or via telephone.

    As you are assessing the woman, the son tells you that he last talked to her the prior evening (approximately 12 hours ago). As you perform a head-tilt chin lift on the patient, you note that her neck is very stiff and difficult to manipulate. She is apneic and pulseless and her skin is pale and cold. You also note that her pupils are fixed and dilated. You note the presence of ecchymosis in dependent areas. The son states that his mother's wishes were to die in peace and at home. He asks you and your partner to honor that by "letting her go" and then presents you with a document that reflects her wishes.

4. What signs have you encountered that would indicate cardiac arrest of a prolonged nature?

    There are multiple signs that this patient has been "down" for a prolonged period of time. First of all, the fact that her neck is stiff and difficult to manipulate indicates rigor mortis, which typically begins within several hours after death. In addition, the patient's skin is cold, indicating a lack of circulation for an extended period of time. The large area of ecchymosis on her back is called lividity, or pooling. As circulation ceases, blood will settle in the areas that are dependent (low) and is very noticeable when these areas are in contact with a flat object (in this case, the bed). *The fixed and dilated pupils indicate severe cerebral anoxia and are not necessarily a sign of obvious death alone; however, they can reinforce the other findings in this particular case. Clearly, from these signs, this patient is obviously deceased and has been for some time.*

You notify medical control and report your findings. The physician advises you not to initiate resuscitation. As you explain this to the son, he sits down and begins to cry. Your partner tends to the son's psychological needs as you begin to make the necessary notifications.

5. How should you and your partner proceed with this situation?

Resuscitative efforts at this point would be futile. Being a case of obvious death, you should follow local protocols including notification of medical control. In addition, law enforcement as well as a medical examiner or coroner should be summoned to the scene. Most states require the presence of law enforcement any time an unattended death has occurred. The EMT cannot "pronounce" a patient dead; only a licensed physician or physician medical examiner can do this. A justice of the peace or coroner will "certify" the patient's death to include the time, date, and any other documentation required in that particular state or locale.

At this point, your concerns should focus on the family. Empathy and support for the family is very important following the loss of a loved one. Even when the family member is expecting the death of a loved one, it is nonetheless a psychological shock when it actually occurs. Explain to the son that resuscitation will not be initiated in accordance with his mother's wishes. If needed, assist the son with any notifications such as other family members or the funeral home. For obvious reasons, if you previously requested back-up personnel, they can be cancelled.

You radio for the police department to respond to the scene, as well as the county medical examiner. In addition, you cancel the responding back-up crew. As your partner is comforting the son, you return your equipment to the ambulance. Upon arrival of the police personnel, you apprise them of the situation.

PATIENT OUTCOME/PATHOPHYSIOLOGY

Due to the obvious signs of death as well as the terminal illness that the patient was suffering from, she was pronounced dead by the physician via telephone at 1758.

Pulselessness and apnea alone do not constitute "obvious" death. You must assess the patient, to including the estimated length of the arrest. This can be accomplished by asking a family member when the patient was last seen alive. In addition to questioning family and bystanders as needed, signs of obvious death to assess for include rigor mortis, lividity, decomposition, decapitation, dismemberment, burned beyond recognition, and open head injury with exposed brain matter. Locally established protocol may delineate other signs of obvious death in addition to those mentioned. If obvious signs of death are not present or the EMT is unsure, resuscitation should begin until ordered to cease by a physician.

1. Which of the following is not considered an "obvious" sign of death, from which the patient cannot be resuscitated?

    a. lividity

    b. pulselessness

    c. rigor mortis

    d. decapitation

2. You are responding to the scene of a major motor vehicle accident. While en route, a law enforcement officer who is already on the scene calls you on the radio and states that the patient is dead. The appropriate action for the EMT based upon this information would be to:

    a. have the dispatcher notify the coroner or medical examiner

    b. turn your lights and siren off and respond code 1 to the scene

    c. proceed as you were until an initial assessment confirms death

    d. notify the dispatcher and advise him that you are returning to service

3. You are performing an initial assessment on an elderly male with an extensive medical history. The patient is pulseless and apneic and his skin cold and dry. You note the presence of rigor mortis in the patient's jaw as well as pooling of blood in the patient's back. You should first:

    a. attach the AED and analyze the patient's rhythm

    b. request the presence of ALS at the scene

    c. notify medical control and report your findings

    d. begin cardiopulmonary resuscitation (CPR) and transport to the hospital where the patient can be pronounced dead

4. The term "lividity" refers to:

    a. stiffness of the patient's joints after death

    b. excessively cold skin indicating prolonged lack of circulation

    c. fixed and dilated pupils that have a glazed appearance to them

    d. settling of the blood to areas of the body that are low or "dependent"

5. A patient in cardiac arrest does not appear to have obvious signs of death; however, his skin is cold to the touch and his pupils are fixed and dilated. The EMT should:

    a. notify medical control prior to initiating CPR

    b. ask the family if a DNR or living will order exists

    c. begin CPR and notify medical control for advice

    d. begin basic life support but do not attach the AED

6. What signs would most likely indicate that a patient has a terminal illness?

    a. multiple medication bottles present in the room

    b. a hospital bed in the patient's room

    c. the fact that the patient has signed a living will

    d. all of these indicate a terminal illness

7. When should resuscitation of a patient not be attempted?

    a. when the family advises you not to

    b. if a police officer orders you not to

    c. if the "down time" of the patient is unknown

    d. when a DNR order has been validated by a physician

8. When summoned to a residence for a "death," an elderly man who states that his wife has passed away and that he does not want you to resuscitate her meets you at the door. What should you do?

    a. notify the police immediately

    b. perform an initial assessment on the patient

    c. honor his wishes and notify the justice of the peace

    d. call medical control prior to initiating any resuscitative efforts

9. An important aspect of the EMT's care at the scene of an obvious death is to:

    a. provide emotional support to the family

    b. have the police question the family

    c. remove the body as soon as possible

    d. check the refrigerator for insulin

10. Who can legally pronounce a patient dead?

    a. an EMT or physician

    b. a physician or police officer

    c. a licensed physician only

    d. a justice of the peace or EMT

2

SHE IS HAVING
A SEIZURE

Objectives

At the conclusion of this scenario, the participant will be able to:

1. Describe the presentation of a patient who has had a seizure.

2. Describe the postictal period following a seizure.

3. List three things that a patient who is refusing care should be told.

SCENARIO

You are called to an office complex for a patient experiencing a seizure. The complex has eight individual buildings arranged in a campus. It could take as long as 7 or 8 minutes to get from the ambulance to the farthest building.

1. How will this impact your size-up and patient care plan?

   It is most important to bring all the equipment you could possibly need with you. This would include, at a minimum, your first-in bag with oxygen, suction, and AED. It would be prudent to put everything on the stretcher and wheel that with you as well; it will give you a means to carry all the equipment. If you think that you will need any help it would be prudent to call for it now. Remember, it will take help a long time to get to you.

   You get to the building that contains the patient and make your way to the sixth floor. The scene appears safe and you are directed to the office containing the patient. You see her leaning against a partition between cubicles. She appears conscious although a bit drowsy. A coworker is kneeling down and reassuring her. "Okay, back to work," she says to a few lingering gawkers.

You introduce yourself to the patient. The woman with her says, "She had a seizure. She is better now." You begin to talk to the patient again and ask her how she is and the coworker interrupts again. "She has a history of seizures. Just give her a minute and she will be okay." Your next question also results in an answer from the woman rather than the patient.

2. How will the coworker's involvement affect patient care? How would you handle this situation?

The coworker means well and has provided important information. It will soon become too much if the patient is never allowed to speak. There could be things the patient would say differently or things she would not want her coworker to hear (e.g., describing incontinence). You could politely tell her that you need the patient to answer for herself or have your partner take her aside to gather more history while you talk to the patient.

You begin to talk to the patient and find that she does indeed have a history of epilepsy. She has seizures occasionally and this one seemed to be of similar duration and type as she usually has. She could see a halo around the lights in the office before she had the seizure. The seizure involved jerking of her extremities and lasted 2 to 3 minutes. As you speak to her you find that she is gradually becoming less sleepy and increasingly oriented. She tells you that she does not want to go to the hospital.

3. What is the significance of seeing the "halo" around lights before the seizure?

It is common for epileptic patients to experience an "aura" before a seizure. This patient experienced a visual aura. Other patients have reported smelling things immediately before a seizure.

4. Why has the patient become less sleepy?

Patients who have a seizure may experience a postictal period. This phase begins with unresponsiveness or extreme drowsiness. The patient gradually becomes more and more responsive until he is alert (or in a normal mental state). Obtaining a history of the events after the seizure will be important in determining the type and cause of seizure.

5. Should this patient refuse treatment?

You will find many seizure patients who do refuse your care and transportation. Patients who have seizures frequently will not go to the hospital each time. Generally, we should try to get patients to go to the hospital. With a seizure where the cause is unknown (a first seizure or in patients who do not have a history of seizures), a serious underlying problem could cause the seizure. Patients who have had status epilepticus in the past should also be urged strongly to go to the hospital. In this case, if it is a type and duration of seizure that the patient frequently has, she may refuse—but only after you offer to treat and transport her and follow your procedures for patient refusal.

Despite your efforts to convince the patient to accept your transportation, she refuses.

6. What must you do now that the patient has refused?

You should be sure that you have told the patient that you are willing to take her to the hospital and that without an examination at the hospital she could have another seizure, this time more serious, possibly resulting in serious injury or death. You should advise her to contact her physician for follow-up and call emergency medical services (EMS) again at any sign of trouble or if she decides to accept transportation at a later time. She should sign a refusal form and a witness should also sign it.

PATIENT OUTCOME/PATHOPHYSIOLOGY

Seizures are defined as a sudden change in sensation, behavior, or movement. In this case there were extreme jerking movements called *convulsions*. Seizures are caused by many things including tumors, infection, metabolic problems, and trauma. The most common cause is a disease called *epilepsy*. Epilepsy may develop after head injury or surgery. Other patients are born with epilepsy.

In this case, the patient recovered fully and experienced no lasting problems from the seizure and refusal of care. She contacted her neurologist who increased her antiseizure medications.

EVALUATION

1. A seizure may exhibit as:
   a. brief loss of consciousness
   b. violent shaking or jerking motions
   c. movement or twitching of an extremity
   d. all of the above

2. Why would you bring your AED to a call for a seizure?
   a. seizure patients frequently go into cardiac arrest
   b. hypoxia from cardiac arrest may cause seizures
   c. seizure calls frequently involve children
   d. AEDs may be used to treat seizures

3. Which of the following statements regarding seizures is FALSE?
   a. Seizure patients must be transported to the hospital.
   b. Seizures may be caused by a prior head injury.
   c. Epilepsy is a disease that causes seizures.
   d. Some seizures manifest only with a vacant stare or brief loss of consciousness.

4. An "aura" describes:
   a. the period of sleepiness after a seizure
   b. minor twitching that accompanies a seizure
   c. an abnormal sensation (e.g. visual, smell) prior to the seizure
   d. a period of fatigue or confusion immediately prior to a seizure

5. Seizures occurring in children without a prior history of seizures are most commonly caused by:
    a. head injury
    b. fever
    c. diabetes
    d. stroke

6. A patient seizing continuously for 9 to 10 minutes is experiencing:
    a. status asthmaticus
    b. Prolonged Neurological Syndrome (PNS)
    c. status epilepticus
    d. febrile seizures

7. Which of the following would indicate that a patient who has experienced a seizure should go to the hospital?
    a. history of seizures
    b. seizure is similar to prior seizures
    c. prolonged seizure
    d. normal mental status following a seizure

8. Which of the following appropriately describes the postictal phase of a seizure?
    a. seizures progressing from rigidity to violent jerking
    b. a period of alertness progressing to unconsciousness
    c. a period of incontinence followed by sleepiness
    d. a period of gradually increasing responsiveness

9. All of the following should be told to a seizure patient who refuses transportation EXCEPT:
    a. another seizure is possible and harm could result from declining transport
    b. the patient should stay with someone if possible
    c. the patient should consider taking additional antiseizure medication
    d. the patient should contact his physician

10. You arrive to find a patient seizing on the floor of a school classroom. Which of the following actions is inappropriate to take?
    a. clear students away from the patient
    b. place a bite stick in the patient's mouth to prevent oral trauma
    c. clear the area of items that could cause harm to the patient
    d. obtain a brief history of the seizure from bystanders

3

UH OH!

Objectives

At the conclusion of this scenario, the participant will be able to:

1. Defend the necessity of reporting medical errors.

2. Describe three points necessary in documenting medical errors.

3. Describe the relation of protocols to prehospital medication administration.

SCENARIO

Your ambulance is dispatched for a patient with severe chest pain. You arrive on a safe scene and find a 68-year-old male patient with a history of high blood pressure who developed chest pain while roller blading. He returned home, where you find him in the kitchen.

The pain is severe and crushing. He holds his fist to his chest in the classic sign of distress. He tells you "I have these here nitro pills." His signs and symptoms match the criteria; his vital signs are adequate. Your medical director has issued you standing orders to use nitroglycerin in cases such as this.

You administer the nitro, which provides considerable relief to the patient. The patient does not have a recurrence of the chest pain and his vitals remain stable en route to the hospital.

When you arrive at the hospital and the driver begins to back into the emergency department your patient says "Thank you for letting me take my wife's nitro. It sure helped. You guys are the best!"

Your heart sinks as you realize that you are allowed to only administer the patient's own nitroglycerin. What you did was a breach of protocol. The patient did not seem to be negatively affected.

1. Do you tell the hospital physician about the nitroglycerin?

   Yes. Absolutely. Unquestionably.

2. What would happen if you tell this physician? If you don't tell the physician?

   You are going to be in some trouble—you violated protocol. But not in as much trouble as you would be if you tried to cover it up.

   In the event of an error your agency will have to take some action. This could range from counseling by the medical director and additional training to more serious actions such as suspension (although this would be rare in events such as this). Protocols are a serious thing. If you tried to cover up an error it would not be unusual to have your certification suspended or revoked and face disciplinary hearings. The difference: dishonesty. EMS involves trust and integrity. We see people at their worst and when they are vulnerable. EMTs must be honest, trustworthy, and act with integrity at all times.

3. Do you document the fact that you gave the patient someone else's nitroglycerin on your prehospital report?

   Yes, although how it is done may vary widely. One option would be to document the call as it happened and to make a note at the end of the narrative that states "Upon arrival at the hospital the patient thanked us for administering the nitro and mentioned that it was his wife's. Dr. (Dr.'s name) was advised immediately upon arrival at the emergency department."

PATIENT OUTCOME/PATHOPHYSIOLOGY

The patient in this scenario had his first episode of angina pectoris that sent up a warning sign: chest pain. He was evaluated in the hospital emergency department and sent upstairs, where it was determined that he had significant blockage of three coronary arteries. He underwent bypass surgery and has returned to an active lifestyle.

The medication administration violated your EMS system's prehospital protocols. The emergency department (ED) physician, your agency's medical director, and administration issued you a letter of warning and directed 16 hours of clinical time in the emergency department working with the nursing staff and learning about medication administration. You were commended for your honesty in reporting the error.

EVALUATION

1. Protocols are defined as:
   a. general guidelines for care
   b. orders given to you by a physician over the radio or cell phone
   c. assessments or interventions to be performed in certain situations
   d. what a reasonable EMT in a similar situation would do

2. You are called to a school playground where a child has been stung by a bee. The patient is blotchy and wheezing. The teacher believes the student is

allergic to bees and offers you another student's epinephrine autoinjector. You should:

    a. allow the teacher to administer the epinephrine

    b. administer the epinephrine yourself

    c. wait for a parent to obtain permission to administer the medication

    d. begin transport and contact medical direction

3. Which one of the following would be a contraindication for nitroglycerin?

    a. chest pain

    b. respiratory distress

    c. blood pressure 90 mmHg

    d. nitroglycerin prescribed to the patient

4. Which of the following is NOT one of the five "rights" of medication administration?

    a. right patient

    b. right route

    c. right dose

    d. right date

    e. right medication

5. All medication errors must be reported.

    a. true

    b. false

6. Making false statements about medication administration or dishonesty in reporting is grounds for revocation of your EMS license or certification.

    a. true

    b. false

7. Which of the following statements about documentation of medical errors is correct?

    a. If you tell the physician verbally you will not need to write a written report.

    b. Written reports are only necessary if harm is done to a patient.

    c. Reports of medication errors should be done factually and objectively.

    d. In most cases medication errors are partially the patient's fault for providing improper information. This should be noted on the report.

8. You administer nitroglycerin to a patient according to your protocols. The patient experiences a sudden, dangerous drop in his blood pressure. This is best described as (a):

    a. medication error

    b. side effect

c. contraindication

d. indication

9. You are treating a patient who meets all of the criteria for administration of nitroglycerin. You are concerned because even though the patient's blood pressure falls within the limits of the protocol it doesn't seem safe to administer the medication. You should:

a. administer the medication because the protocols have been met

b. administer the medication and document any negative effects

c. contact medical direction for advice

d. not administer the medication and transport the patient

10. You are called to a diabetic patient who is unresponsive. You have oral glucose available. The patient meets all of the protocol requirements except that the unconscious patient should not receive anything by mouth. You should:

a. give tiny amounts of glucose that the patient won't aspirate

b. ask the family member to administer glucose since you are not able to

c. transport the patient with oxygen

d. administer oxygen and wait for him to regain consciousness, give glucose, and transport

4

I CAN'T BREATHE

Objectives

At the conclusion of this scenario, the participant will be able to:

1. Perform an organized assessment on a patient with a respiratory complaint.

2. Recognize the signs and symptoms of acute respiratory insufficiency and failure.

3. Understand the principles of both initial and ongoing management modalities for the patient with respiratory compromise.

SCENARIO

You are dispatched to a residence for a patient with difficulty breathing. The time is 1745 and the scene is approximately 10 minutes from your station.

1. What are your thought processes as you are responding to the scene?

In addition to driving the ambulance with due regard for those around you, you may be thinking that a patient who complains of respiratory distress could be experiencing a number of problems such as hyperventilation syndrome, acute myocardial infarction, anaphylaxis, asthma, bronchitis, pneumothorax, pneumonia, or acute pulmonary embolism, to name a few. Additionally, you should be concerned with the setting in which this emergency took place. You do not have enough information yet to be able to determine whether or not this is a medical case or whether the patient was injured, perhaps by an individual who may still be in the area; therefore, scene safety should be at the forefront of your mind.

With your estimated time of arrival (ETA) to the scene being 8 minutes, the dispatcher notifies you that the patient has called back in a panicked, broken voice, begging you to hurry up. Upon arrival, you perform a scene size-up and note that the patient is an approximately 64-year-old man nervously pacing in his front yard. The scene is otherwise safe to enter.

The patient states: "I was watching TV and suddenly, I could not catch my breath. I had to get out of the house to get some fresh air."

2. What have you learned about the patient from the general impression, his chief complaint, as well as the preliminary portion of your initial assessment?

Your general impression of the patient should be that of one who is restless (pacing in the yard), perhaps due to hypoxia. His chief complaint of difficulty breathing could certainly be a causative factor to hypoxia. An acute onset of respiratory distress should narrow things down a bit for you. Possible causes of a sudden onset of breathing difficulty include acute hyperventilation syndrome, spontaneous pneumothorax, acute asthma attack, acute myocardial infarction, and acute pulmonary embolism.

As you continue your initial assessment of the patient, you note that he is in a considerable degree of respiratory distress. His airway is clear and respirations are adequate although labored. His radial pulse is weak and rapid and his skin is somewhat cool and moist to the touch. His restlessness makes your assessment difficult. As you make a quick visual glance over his entire body, you note that his jugular veins appear distended. There are no other obvious abnormalities that you can see.

3. What significant findings have you discovered in the initial assessment? What might they indicate?

The patient's minimal word sentences mark the severity of his distress. A pulse that is weak and rapid as well as cool, moist skin are all signs of hypoperfusion (shock). Again, the fact that he is restless should reinforce your suspicion of hypoxia. Jugular venous distention (JVD) could indicate a variety of problems. Your assessment is not complete enough at this point to equate the JVD to any one underlying cause.

4. What are your priorities of management based upon your findings thus far?

Oxygen, and lots of it! This patient is painting you a perfect picture of impending respiratory failure. You must ensure the delivery of 100 percent oxygen. Additionally, assisted ventilation may become necessary should the patient's breathing become inadequate. Due to the potential of deterioration, rapid transport to the hospital is indicated. Any patient with a hypoxic event is at risk of cardiopulmonary arrest; therefore, an AED should be readily available.

You ask your partner to place the patient on 100 percent oxygen via nonrebreather mask and to obtain a set of baseline vital signs as you perform a rapid exam of the patient. The results of these findings are as follows:

Baseline vital signs
- Blood pressure of 98/60, pulse of 120/weak, respirations labored at a rate of 28

Rapid exam
- Jugular venous distention
- Diminished breath sounds to the right side of the chest

You place the patient onto the stretcher and position him in a full-fowler position. The patient tells you that he wishes to be transported to a hospital in a nearby town, which is approximately 30 miles away, despite the fact that there is a closer facility within 12 miles of the scene.

5. Are you comfortable with the patient's choice of hospitals, with regard to the transport time? If not, what would be your recommendation(s) to the patient?

You should be very uncomfortable transporting a hypoxic patient for 30 miles. Generally, we should transport our patients to the hospital of their choice. In this case, you should explain the situation to the patient and request that he allow you to transport him to the closer facility. Your locally established protocols should provide guidance for hospital diversion in select patients. If you are unsure, contact medical control for advice. If the patient maintains his choice of hospitals, the physician may wish to speak to the patient over the phone to ensure that he understands the seriousness of the situation.

As you begin transport, you obtain a SAMPLE (S–Signs and Symptoms; A–Allergies; M–Medications; P–Pertinent Past history; L–Last oral intake; E–Events leading up to the injury or illness) history from the patient. He tells you that he is allergic to penicillin and is presently taking Motrin for a minor back injury that has kept him in bed for the past three days. His past medical history is significant for hypertension. He can't remember when he last ate, and the preceding events were that he was watching TV at the onset of symptoms.

6. What components of the SAMPLE history put this patient at risk for a respiratory problem?

- *With an allergy to penicillin, you must ensure that the patient did not inadvertently take a derivative of this medication (amoxicillin, dicloxacillin, etc.), which would result in an allergic reaction. In addition, many patients are told that they are allergic to ibuprofen but don't realize that medications such as Motrin, Advil, and Nuprin all contain ibuprofen as the active ingredient.*
- *A history of hypertension is a risk factor for acute myocardial infarction, congestive heart failure with pulmonary edema, and acute pulmonary embolism. Also, the patient does not take any medications to control his high blood pressure, so uncontrolled hypertension puts him at an even higher risk.*
- *Due to the patient's back injury, he has been at prolonged bed rest. This is a significant risk factor for the development of an embolism, which could travel to and lodge in a pulmonary artery. As the patient remains supine for prolonged periods of time, blood in the lower extremities tends to stagnate. As a result, the formation of a thrombus (clot) could break loose and travel to other parts of the body (embolism).*

7. What is the explanation for this patient's rapid deterioration?

This patient is now in respiratory failure (shock) and impending respiratory arrest. His respirations of 30 and shallow mark his failing respiratory system. An absent radial pulse indicates significant hypotension, which is a late sign of shock. The weak carotid pulse reinforces the significance of his hypotension. The cyanosis that is developing, which is a later sign of respiratory failure, indicates a severe lack of oxygen in the patient's arterial blood.

With an estimated time of arrival at the hospital of 7 minutes, you are performing an ongoing assessment of the patient and note that his level of consciousness is markedly decreased. You immediately repeat the initial assessment and find that his respirations are now 30 and shallow; his radial pulse is absent with a carotid pulse weak at a rate of 140. In addition, you note that he is developing cyanosis around his lips.

8. How will your management differ now as opposed to initially?

Supplemental oxygen is no longer sufficient for this patient because the mechanics of his breathing will not allow for the adequate uptake of the oxygen. You must reassess and ensure a patent airway, either with an oropharyngeal airway should he become unconscious and lose his gag reflex or a nasopharyngeal airway if he remains semiconscious. Positive pressure ventilation via either a pocket mask with supplemental oxygen or bag-valve mask device must be initiated immediately. Suction must be readily available should the patient begin to vomit. Do not forget the AED! This patient is extremely close to full cardiac arrest.

Since you are busy managing the deteriorating patient, you tell your partner to notify the hospital of your impending arrival, which is less than 5 minutes away. You deliver the patient, who is now unconscious, to the hospital and transfer care to the attending emergency department physician.

PATIENT OUTCOME/PATHOPHYSIOLOGY

The patient was received at the emergency department and was immediately intubated. He was diagnosed with an acute pulmonary embolism, managed with aggressive ventilatory support, and given a blood-thinning medication called Heparin in an attempt to dissolve the lodged embolism. After a stay in the hospital of 2 weeks, the patient was discharged home. Your medical director commends you and your partner on your thorough assessment and aggressive management of the patient.

A pulmonary embolism, which is the blockage of a pulmonary artery by either a blood clot or air, prevents the blood from being oxygenated in the lungs and leads to severe hypoxia. As the pulmonary artery becomes blocked, blood backs up into the right side of the heart and eventually into the systemic circulation. Jugular venous distention indicates this backing up of blood. As the lungs do not receive oxygen, the alveoli begin to collapse (atelectasis), which causes a diminishing in breath sounds. Major risk factors for a pulmonary embolism include hypertension (especially uncontrolled hypertension), prolonged bed rest, and recent surgery. Recall that this patient had two of these significant risk factors.

1. While assessing a conscious patient complaining of respiratory distress, you note that the patient has stopped talking to you. You should:

   a. ensure a patent airway and assist breathing

   b. assess for a carotid and radial pulse

   c. increase the amount of oxygen delivery

   d. assess the patient's responsiveness

2. Early signs of hypoxia in the adult patient include:

   a. cool, dry skin

   b. a weak, slow pulse

   c. restlessness or anxiety

   d. unconsciousness

3. While delivering oxygen to a patient with a nonrebreather mask, the patient becomes very restless and pulls the mask from his face, yet he remains conscious and alert. The appropriate management for this situation would be to:

   a. begin assisting ventilations with a bag-valve mask

   b. ensure that you have the flowmeter set at 15 liters/min

   c. place the patient on a nasal cannula at 1–6 liters/min

   d. tell the patient he needs the oxygen and tape the mask to his face

4. Which of the following combinations of airway devices are typically used for an unconscious patient with inadequate breathing?

   a. an oropharyngeal airway and nonrebreather

   b. a nasopharyngeal airway and a pocket mask

   c. an oropharyngeal airway and bag-valve mask

   d. a nasopharyngeal airway and nasal cannula

5. During respiratory failure, patients lose consciousness secondary to:

   a. a significantly fast heart rate

   b. a lack of oxygen to the brain

   c. a lack of carbon dioxide in the blood

   d. severe anxiety caused by the respiratory distress

6. A 45-year-old male calls EMS because he is experiencing severe difficulty breathing that began approximately 2 hours ago. The EMT's initial action should be to:

   a. assess the patient's airway

   b. apply 100 percent oxygen to the patient

   c. form a general impression of the patient

   d. auscultate the patient's breath sounds

7. A patient complaining of respiratory difficulty suddenly loses consciousness. The EMT should immediately:

    a. begin assisting ventilations

    b. repeat the initial assessment

    c. assess for the presence of a pulse

    d. place the patient in the recovery position

8. While ventilating a nonbreathing patient he begins to vomit. The EMT should first:

    a. suction the patient's oropharynx

    b. insert an oropharyngeal airway

    c. place the patient on his side to facilitate drainage

    d. continue ventilations while providing oral suctioning

9. After completing the action on the patient in question 8, you should:

    a. suction the patient's oropharynx

    b. insert an oropharyngeal airway

    c. place the patient on his side to facilitate drainage

    d. continue ventilations while providing oral suctioning

10. A patient with a sudden onset of respiratory distress is least likely to be experiencing:

    a. pulmonary embolism

    b. pneumonia

    c. spontaneous pneumothorax

    d. acute myocardial infarction

5

DIFFICULTY BREATHING

Objectives

At the conclusion of this scenario, the participant will be able to:

1. Perform an organized assessment on a patient with a respiratory complaint.

2. Recognize the signs and symptoms of an acute asthma attack.

3. Understand the pathophysiology of asthma.

4. Understand the principles of management, including the use of prescribed inhalers for the patient suffering an acute asthma attack.

SCENARIO

At 0430, your team is dispatched to a convenience store. Apparently, the clerk called 911 in a voice indicating obvious respiratory distress and requested EMS. He then hung up the phone. The temperature outside is approximately 30 degrees with the winds blowing at 25 miles per hour. Your response time to the scene is approximately 6 minutes.

1. Are there any peculiarities about this call that you are thinking about while you are en route to the scene?

   You can never be sure of what you are actually responding to. The season seems appropriate for an influx of patients with breathing problems; however, given the odd circumstances of the call you cannot discount the possibility that the clerk may be actually a panicked caller who is being robbed. You should notify the police and have them respond to the scene prior to your arrival.

You arrive on scene at 0436, shortly after the police, where you encounter a 25-year-old male inside the store. You can see through the window of the store that a patron has the patient breathing into a paper bag. The police officer motions for you to come inside.

2. What is your initial reaction based upon your rather vague general impression of the patient?

The paper bag has to go! It is no longer a standard of care to "rebreathe" patients into a paper bag; even if it appears that they are having an anxiety attack. The standard of care is to verbally coach the patient to slow his breathing and apply oxygen. It is still public perception that bag rebreathing is an effective treatment when in reality it can be extremely detrimental to the patient. If this patient is hyperventilating due to problems such as diabetic ketoacidosis or hypoxia, he needs to be provided 100 percent oxygen, not his own exhaled carbon dioxide.

Upon initial assessment, you note that the patient's airway is open but he is having severe difficulty breathing and you can hear audible wheezing both on inhalation and exhalation. As you auscultate his chest, you hear wheezes in all lung fields. The patient states, in two-word sentences, that he has asthma and that this is probably the worst attack that he can remember. He tells you that he had to be in the hospital on a ventilator for this same problem approximately 6 months ago. Upon further assessment, you note that his heart rate is palpable at the wrist at a bounding rate of 130. The pulse oximeter reads 85 percent on room air so you direct your partner to place the patient on 100 percent oxygen with a nonrebreather mask. The remainder of the initial assessment is unremarkable.

3. What is significant about your findings in the initial assessment and the information that he has provided you with?

There are several significant aspects of the initial assessment as well as the information that the patient has provided to you. First of all, a patient with "severe" respiratory distress and minimal word sentences in and of itself indicates a severe respiratory problem. Second, the fact that the patient is an asthmatic and has been on a ventilator before indicates that he has a history of status asthmaticus; therefore, you should be prepared to potentially assist the ventilations of the patient. The tachycardia can be due to a variety of factors, from fear to hypoxia. With a room-air oxygen saturation of 85 percent, it is obvious that the patient is hypoxic. Wheezing on both inhalation and exhalation indicates a severe asthma attack.

As you direct your partner to go to the ambulance to get the stretcher, you obtain a baseline set of vital signs as well as a SAMPLE history. Your findings are as follows:

Baseline vital signs
- Blood pressure—140/90
- Pulse—130 and bounding
- Respirations—30 and labored with audible wheezing

SAMPLE history
- S—severe difficulty breathing and audible wheezing
- A—pollen and dust

- M—Albuterol inhaler and Vanceril inhaler
- P—asthma, recent upper-respiratory infection, appendectomy
- L—approximately 6 hours ago, dinner before coming to work
- E—he was reading a newspaper when the symptoms began

4. What additional questions might you ask the patient that you haven't already covered in the SAMPLE history?

You should ask the patient if a physician prescribed the Albuterol inhaler to him and if so, whether or not he has taken any puffs from that inhaler prior to your arrival. NOTE: Albuterol is the choice medication prescribed to patients with asthma, bronchitis, and other reactive airway diseases. It is a smooth muscle relaxant (the bronchioles are smooth muscles) and thereby results in bronchodilation when administered. Other names for Albuterol are Ventolin and Proventil.

Vanceril is the brand name of an inhaled steroid. You will find many asthma patients on this or a similar medication. The steroid reduces inflammation in the respiratory tract and prevents attacks. If a patient is having an asthma attack be sure that you are using the correct medication: the bronchodilator and not the inhaled steroid. Steroids are effective for long-term prevention only and do not help in emergency situations.

5. Are there any identifiable factors about his recent history as well as the present situation that could trigger an asthma attack?

There are several potential causes of this patient's asthma attack in this particular case. A recent history of an upper-respiratory tract infection is a very common factor that tends to precipitate an asthma attack. Also, he is allergic to pollen and dust and if you will recall, the temperature is 30 degrees, which indicates a cold front. Patients with respiratory problems tend to emerge any time the temperature changes, especially from warm to cold. The wind blowing at 30 miles per hour would most definitely kick up any dust as well as pollen from the trees, both of which the patient is allergic to.

After loading the patient into the ambulance, you connect the nonrebreather to the on-board oxygen supply and notify medical control. Your partner is talking to the patient in an attempt to gather further information. The patient states that he only took one puff from his inhaler prior to EMS arrival.

6. When you notify medical control of the situation, what questions and orders should you expect to receive?

You can expect that the physician will want to ensure that the Albuterol is indeed prescribed to him. In addition, he will inquire as to whether or not he took any puffs from that inhaler prior to your arrival. Since the inhaler is prescribed to the patient and he only took one puff, the physician will most likely order you to assist the patient in taking up to two more puffs from the inhaler. NOTE: If the inhaler is not prescribed to the patient, is expired, and/or he has taken up to three puffs prior to your arrival, additional doses of Albuterol are not indicated unless requested by medical control. Medications such as Albuterol cause bronchodilation, thereby enhancing the movement of air through the bronchioles. Common side effects of the medication include anxiety, tachycardia, and coughing.

Remember the five "rights" of medication administration:

- Right patient
- Right medication
- Right time
- Right dose
- Right route

After rendering the care ordered by the physician, the patient's respiratory distress improves significantly and he is now able to talk in full sentences. You begin transport of the patient to the facility that he requests, which is approximately 15 minutes away. En route, you notify the receiving facility of the 10–15 minute estimated time of arrival with a 25-year-old asthmatic, who after treatment is much improved from when you first arrived at the scene. In addition, you advise the facility that the patient's vital signs are stable and that he is on 100 percent oxygen via nonrebreather. The patient is delivered to the emergency department in stable condition.

PATIENT OUTCOME/PATHOPHYSIOLOGY

After a 3-hour stay in the emergency department, it was determined that the patient suffered an acute asthma attack, most likely due to several factors. Since he was in no respiratory distress in the emergency department and the pulse oximeter read 98 percent on room air, he was discharged home with a refill for his Albuterol.

Asthma is a disease with an onset that tends to occur at an early age; however, it can occur later in life as well. It is an episodic reactive airway disease that results in constriction of the bronchioles in the lungs, which explains the wheezing or whistling sound heard when the patient is having an attack. This leads to a decrease in the ability of the patient to effectively breathe and ultimately results in hypoxia due to the interruption of oxygen and carbon dioxide exchange in the lungs. The most severe asthma attack is called status asthmaticus, which results from severe, widespread bronchoconstriction with little or no air movement. Status asthmaticus is a life-threatening situation. Common precipitating factors of an asthma attack include a recent upper-airway infection, allergies, emotional stress, and changes in temperature. The goal in managing asthma is to relieve bronchoconstriction and to improve ventilation.

EVALUATION

1. Which of the following medications is another name for Albuterol?
   a. Alupent
   b. Bronkosol
   c. Atrovent
   d. Proventil

2. A young female with a history of asthma presents with an acute onset of shortness of breath. She is alert and oriented, speaking full sentences. When you auscultate breath sounds, you hear scattered wheezing on exhalation. She is suffering from:

    a. a mild asthma attack

    b. a moderate asthma attack

    c. a severe asthma attack

    d. status asthmaticus

3. Typical precursors to an asthma attack include all of the following EXCEPT:

    a. emotional stress

    b. an ear infection

    c. a respiratory infection

    d. changes in temperature

4. You respond to the residence of a 42-year-old female who complains of difficulty breathing. As you are assessing her, she tells you that she has asthma. Her neighbor, who suffers from asthma as well, has given her an Albuterol inhaler and the patient asks you to assist her in taking the medication. This situation should be managed by:

    a. assisting her in taking the medication because you know it is indicated, then notifying medical control

    b. obtaining a signed release form from the neighbor giving permission to use her medication

    c. placing the patient on a nasal cannula at 4 liters per minute and assisting her in taking the medication if she does not improve

    d. administering oxygen via nonrebreather mask and contacting medical control for advice

5. Prior to administering a prescribed inhaler, the EMT should:

    a. ensure that the inhaler is not expired

    b. make sure the medication is prescribed to the patient

    c. obtain physician permission to assist with the inhaler

    d. do all of these prior to administering an inhaler

6. An asthmatic patient is semiconscious with shallow respirations. She has a prescribed Albuterol inhaler. Which of the following is a priority in the management of this patient?

    a. assisting her in taking the prescribed inhaler

    b. obtaining physician permission to administer the medication

    c. ensuring an adequate airway and assisting ventilations as needed

    d. ensuring an adequate airway and placing the patient on a nonrebreather mask

7. Select the true statement with regards to the pathophysiology of asthma.
   a. The underlying problem with asthma is bronchodilation.
   b. Constriction of the bronchioles results in wheezing.
   c. Dilation of the bronchioles results in wheezing.
   d. Wheezing on both inhalation and expiration indicates a mild attack.

8. Which of the following is not a common side effect of prescribed inhalers such as Albuterol?
   a. bradycardia
   b. tachycardia
   c. anxiety
   d. coughing

9. What information with regards to an asthmatic patient's past medical history should alert the EMT to the potential seriousness of the situation?
   a. the patient is allergic to pollen and molds
   b. the patient has an average of two attacks per year
   c. the patient has been placed on a ventilator in the past
   d. the patient has been seen by a physician two times in the last month

10. The ultimate goal in managing the patient with an acute asthma attack is to:
    a. relieve bronchodilation and increase oxygenation
    b. make the patient comfortable and administer oxygen
    c. reverse the bronchoconstriction and improve breathing
    d. identify whether or not the patient has a prescribed inhaler

6

IT IS HARD TO BREATHE

Objectives

At the conclusion of this scenario, the participant will be able to:

1. Describe the pathophysiology of chronic obstructive pulmonary disease (COPD).

2. List common causes of acute difficulty with breathing.

3. Identify signs and symptoms of COPD exacerbation.

SCENARIO

Your EMS unit is dispatched to the home of an adult male with difficulty breathing. The home is less than 5 minutes from your station.

1. What are your thoughts regarding the dispatch information?

   Your dispatch information is limited. Difficulty breathing in an adult may have many causes. Trauma has not been ruled out so it must remain a potential cause. If trauma is not the issue then many medical causes must be considered. Some of these causes include: asthma, pneumonia, spontaneous pneumothorax, bronchitis, emphysema, and toxic inhalation. More information is needed, as well as your assessment findings, before a potential cause may be identified.

2. What do you do before exiting your ambulance?

   You must gather your personal protective equipment for body substance isolation. This should include, as a minimum, gloves and eye protection. Many patients with medical problems leading to difficulty breathing may be coughing. Coughing is a leading cause of spread of infection by "droplet" form.

As you approach the scene you must be very observant for scene safety. Although the dispatch information may lead you to believe that this is a medical call, you must be aware that EMS services have been dispatched to violent situations in which the caller reports a "medical problem" to avoid law enforcement response. Ensure your safety during all phases of EMS response, care, and transportation.

You arrive at the residence where, at the front door, you are met by the patient's wife. She informs you that her husband is 60 years old and he has emphysema from years of smoking. He wears oxygen and takes numerous medications. His difficulty breathing has progressively gotten worse throughout the day.

3. What have you learned from this bystander information?

Emphysema is a form of chronic obstructive pulmonary disease (COPD). It is characterized by gradual destruction of the alveolar structure. The alveoli become hardened and are therefore restricted from expanding and recoiling. Along with this loss of mobility the interface between the alveoli and the pulmonary capillaries is impeded. It becomes more difficult for oxygen to cross the alveolar wall and enter into the blood system. Waste products in the blood, such as CO_2, also begin to build up because they cannot cross the alveolar membrane to be exhaled.

This patient is also on home-oxygen therapy. This is a very advanced stage of COPD. In many medical patients the administration of oxygen oftentimes allows EMS personnel to see a dramatic improvement in symptoms. However, this may not be the case with this patient.

You are directed into the living room. You find the patient sitting bolt upright in a recliner. You can see that he is wearing a nasal cannula. He is utilizing accessory muscles to breath. You also witness the patient performing "pursed lip" breathing. On the table, next to the patient, you see two bottles of medication, along with one inhaler. You also see several Kleenexes that have been utilized.

4. What are your thoughts regarding these findings from across the room?

You will need to ascertain how much oxygen the patient is receiving. The use of accessory muscles indicates that the patient is displaying signs of respiratory distress. This should alert you that this is a serious situation, one that may require a short scene time. Pursed lip breathing is very common in COPD patients. They "purse" or tighten their lips during exhalation in an attempt to generate a "higher" pressure within their lungs. This helps to expand their alveoli and, it is hoped, improve oxygenation. The significance of the Kleenex is that the patient is probably coughing up a lot of phlegm. This may indicate that the patient is suffering from a pulmonary infection such as pneumonia. This may be the cause of this exacerbation of his COPD.

You introduce yourself to the patient and ascertain his permission to assess and treat him. Your immediate assessment reveals that the patient is awake and alert. His airway is open with mild to moderate respiratory distress. No cyanosis is evident. You palpate a radial pulse which is rapid at 120/minute and bounding. You begin to gather information for your focused history. You note that the patient is having difficulty speaking in complete sentences. He reports to you that he is on oxygen at 1½ Lpm. He noted that he actually began to get worse last night because he was coughing and was bringing up thick, yellow-colored phlegm. Today the phlegm is thicker and more of a brown color. He didn't sleep very well during the night because of his coughing and his worsening dyspnea. When asked about his medical history he reports that he has a history of heart problems, along with his emphysema. He takes Digoxin daily for his heart and was started 3 weeks ago on a medication called Prednisone. He also uses an inhaler called Combivent four times a day.

5. What is the importance of brown-colored phlegm?

This patient's phlegm has changed color, from yellow to brown. Brown-colored sputum often signifies a bacterial infection. Many by-products of bacterial growth and replication cause body fluids to darken. Pneumonia may be a cause.

6. Do you recognize these medications?

Digoxin (aka: Lanoxin) is a common heart medication used for heart failure. It causes the heart to beat in a more regular rhythm and also causes a more forceful contraction.
     Prednisone (aka: Novoprednisone) is known as a corticosteroid. It is used to decrease inflammation, in this case, within the lungs. It may be useful when a patient has diffuse pulmonary inflammation causing an exacerbation of symptoms. One of the side effects, however, is that it decreases the body's ability to fight infection. This medication may have facilitated bacterial growth in the lungs.
     Combivent (aka: Combination Atrovent and Albuterol) is an inhaled bronchodilator. It allows distal airways to relax, opening the lumen for air exchange. It is usually prescribed in a hand-held inhaler.

You direct your partner to obtain vital signs, including a pulse oximeter reading, as you begin your focused physical exam. You note that the patient is very thin with a "barrel chest." The airway remains open and patent. Breathing remains moderately labored. Intercostal muscle use is evident. Auscultation of breath sounds reveals bilateral expiratory wheezes in all lobes. Some coarse rhonchi sounds are heard in both lower bases. The abdomen is soft. The extremities are normal with palpable pulses and good sensory and motor function. Pupils are equal, round, and reactive to light. Your partner reports the following vital signs: B/P 148/90, HR 120, RR 22, and an SpO_2 reading of 89 percent on 1½ Lpm oxygen.

7. Why is the patient very thin?

Patients with chronic lung disease have a higher metabolic rate than normal patients. Their body is basically in "overdrive" to meet the demands of the respiratory system. Many patients do not eat very well because it interrupts their efforts to breath or because they have an altered sense of taste. They simply do not ingest enough calories to meet their body's needs.

8. What is the significance of a barrel chest appearance?

Emphysema patients often develop a barrel chest appearance because they have stagnant air trapped in their alveoli. The lungs are basically overdistended.

9. What will you do for an SpO_2 of 89 percent?

This patient is already on oxygen at 1½ Lpm. The first action would be to simply increase the oxygen to 3 or 4 Lpm. This is acceptable because the patient is in mild to moderate distress. We may then monitor for improvement before giving higher concentrations of oxygen.

You direct your partner to connect the nasal cannula to your portable device at 3 Lpm. Your partner begins to prepare the stretcher as you gather your SAMPLE history. The patient states that his symptoms began last night as he described earlier. He denies allergies to medications. He only takes the three medicines you saw on the table. He admits to a past medical history of emphysema and heart failure. He last ate broth 2 hours ago. He took some more of his Combivent inhaler just before you arrived on scene.

10. Why wouldn't you start oxygen at a higher flow?

> We never withhold oxygen from someone who needs it. However, patients with COPD may have an altered process of breathing control. You and I regulate our breathing by how much build up of CO_2 we have during exertion. A patient with COPD regulates his breathing by how low his oxygen gets. Therefore, if we give too much oxygen to a patient with COPD, he may actually stop breathing because his brain tells his body it has enough oxygen. If you are required to give high concentrations of oxygen to a patient with COPD for reasons such as trauma, altered mental status, severe distress, or cyanosis you must be immediately ready to assist ventilations with a bag-valve mask if he stops breathing.

You assist the patient to the stretcher, where he is secured with head of the stretcher elevated. He is continued on oxygen at 3 Lpm. You see an improvement of his SpO_2 to 94 percent, as well as an improvement in his respiratory distress. You instruct the wife to bring his medications with her to the hospital, as she states she will be driving herself there. You place the patient in the ambulance and begin the 7-minute ride to the hospital. Your patient continues to improve and tolerates the transport without incident. You deliver your patient to the hospital where you give a verbal and written report to the hospital personnel.

PATIENT OUTCOME/PATHOPHYSIOLOGY

Your patient is admitted to the hospital for several days with the diagnosis of acute exacerbation of COPD secondary to pneumonia. He was treated with IV antibiotics and he was taken off of the Prednisone therapy. He was discharged to home where he will continue to need oxygen therapy.

You are very aware that there is no cure for emphysema and that his condition will continue to deteriorate. You fully expect to respond to this man's house again in the future.

EVALUATION

1. Which of the following is the greatest risk factor for the onset of emphysema?
   a. asthma
   b. CHF
   c. smoking
   d. cystic fibrosis

2. Which of the following must be avoided in the house of a patient utilizing home oxygen?

a. water soluble lubricants
b. open flame
c. AEDs
d. occlusive dressings

3. Inhalers are utilized by patients for which of the following reasons?

a. dilate bronchioles
b. constrict bronchioles
c. decrease phlegm production
d. increase oxygen-hemoglobin binding

4. Which of the following are signs of exacerbation of COPD?

a. thickened, discolored phlegm
b. increased use of accessory muscles
c. increased work of breathing
d. all of the above

5. The medical term for difficulty breathing is:

a. apnea
b. lethargia
c. dyspnea
d. dentitia

6. COPD patients who complain of difficulty breathing should always be started on oxygen at 15 Lpm with a nonrebreather mask.

a. true
b. false

7. Chronic air trapping in the lungs, along with increased use of chest muscles to breath, may lead to which of the following:

a. barrel chest appearance
b. pursed-lip breathing
c. a thin, wasting, appearance
d. all of the above

8. Coarse lung sounds caused by fluid or phlegm in the distal airways are termed:

a. wheezes
b. rales
c. rhonchi
d. stridor

9. Musical sounds caused by constriction of the distal airways are termed:
    a. wheezes
    b. rales
    c. rhonchi
    d. stridor

10. Digoxin is a medication used for the treatment of:
    a. emphysema
    b. chronic bronchitis
    c. congestive heart failure
    d. low potassium levels

7

UNCONSCIOUS MALE

Objectives

At the conclusion of this scenario, the participant will be able to:

1. Relate the integration of the AED with the management of a cardiac arrest patient.

2. Explain the importance of early defibrillation in the cardiac arrest patient.

3. Define the indications and contraindications for the use of the automated external defibrillator (AED).

SCENARIO

At 1650, your unit gets dispatched to the scene of an "unconscious male." The location of the incident is less than 2 minutes from your station. You arrive on scene at 1653, where you find a male who is approximately 50 years of age lying in a supine position in his front yard. A neighbor is providing one-rescuer CPR on the patient, who was witnessed to have collapsed approximately 3 minutes earlier. Your partner immediately notifies the dispatcher and requests an ALS unit.

1. With this particular patient, what has "set the stage" for a potentially successful resuscitation?

   There are a multitude of factors that are going to maximize the chances of a successful resuscitation. In this case they include:

   - Early access: It is obvious from the patient's "down time" of only 3 minutes that EMS was notified immediately. This is the first link in the "chain of survival."

- Early CPR: The second link in the chain of survival is early CPR. The neighbor has apparently witnessed the cardiac arrest and provided immediate CPR. Timely and adequate CPR will keep this patient's heart and brain oxygenated until EMS arrives.
- Early defibrillation (your short response time): Since it only took you 2 minutes to arrive at the scene, this patient will receive early defibrillation if needed, which has clearly been documented as being the most important factor in the resuscitation of cardiac arrest patients.
- Early ALS intervention: The fact that your partner requested an advanced life support unit immediately upon arrival will allow this patient to receive treatment such as advanced airway support and medication therapy that the EMT cannot provide.

As you can see, all four links in the American Heart Association's "chain of survival" are intact; therefore, this patient stands an excellent chance of being resuscitated.

You and your partner exit the ambulance, grab your medical kit and AED, and proceed to the patient's side. Once there, your partner asks the neighbor to stop CPR while he verifies pulselessness and apnea.

2. Why verify the fact that the patient is pulseless and apneic when CPR is obviously in progress?

It is important for the EMT to perform an initial assessment on all patients. Many times, patients have CPR unnecessarily performed because they actually had a pulse and were unconscious from a cause other than cardiac arrest (i.e. hypoglycemia, drug ingestion, etc.). Unnecessary CPR can cause further harm to the patient. Remember the first rule of medicine, "First, do no harm."

3. As your partner is assessing the patient, what should your initial actions be focused on, and why?

Getting the AED ready! It is estimated that 75 percent of cardiac arrest patients present with ventricular fibrillation (V-Fib) as the initial cardiac rhythm. The AED is designed to shock this rhythm. The patient may also be in ventricular tachycardia (V-Tach) without a pulse, which the AED will shock as well. For each minute that ventricular fibrillation or pulseless ventricular tachycardia remains untreated, there is 10 percent less likelihood that the patient will be successfully resuscitated. Prolonged hypoxia from cardiac arrest will result in the production of a chemical called lactic acid. This combination of hypoxia and lactic acid will rapidly deteriorate the patient's rhythm to asystole, after which time the chances of survival are dismal.

Your partner verifies that the patient is pulseless and apneic. He assists the neighbor in performing two-rescuer CPR as you ready the defibrillator. You direct your partner and the neighbor to temporarily stop CPR while you attach the AED pads to the patient's chest in order to analyze his cardiac rhythm.

4. Describe the correct placement of the AED pads on the patient's chest.

There are two (2) pads that must be applied to the patient's chest. The white (negative) pad is placed to the right of the upper sternum and the red (positive) pad is placed over the lower left ribs. Alternatively, the pads can be placed in the anterior-posterior position, with the white pad being placed on the front directly over the heart and the red pad placed on the back directly under the left scapula. It is important to note that some AEDs will not function correctly with this alternative pad placement; therefore, the EMT must be familiar with the type of AED being used.

5. What else must be evaluated prior to analysis of the patient's cardiac rhythm?

You must ensure that the pads are securely adhered to the patient's chest, without any air pockets in between the pad and the patient's chest. Air pockets will result in burns to the patient's chest and a less effective defibrillation. Additionally, you must make sure that the patient is not wet or laying in water. This poses a direct threat to rescuer safety! If needed, the patient must be rapidly moved from the water and/or his chest dried off prior to placement of the pads. Since the AED will not analyze the rhythm of a patient that is moving, all contact with the patient must cease.

6. What safety procedures are taken prior to defibrillation?

Whoever is operating the AED must ensure that nobody is in contact with the patient prior to performing defibrillation. This involves not only verbalizing "clear," but visual confirmation as well.

*   This occurs for each of the subsequent shocks. After the first defibrillation is delivered, the AED automatically reanalyzes the cardiac rhythm. This function of the AED emphasizes the importance of rapidly identifying and defibrillating the rhythm if necessary. The AED delivers shocks in sets of three. The initial three shocks are delivered at 200, 300, and 360 joules, respectively. After the first three initial shocks have been delivered, further defibrillations will be delivered at 360 joules.*

After correctly placing the pads on the patient's chest, you turn the AED on and tell your partner and the neighbor to "stand clear" as you press the analyze button. After a brief period, you see a message stating "shock advised." After the capacitor in the AED is charged, the "shock" light illuminates. After ensuring that nobody is in contact with the patient, you press the discharge button and deliver the first defibrillation. The AED immediately goes back into the analyze mode.

After the AED reanalyzes the patient's rhythm, it again advises the need for a shock. You repeat the defibrillation procedure, after which the AED autoanalyzes again. However, this time it advises you to "check pulse." You assess the carotid pulse and note that it has returned. The ALS ambulance is approximately 5 minutes away.

7. If the patient had not resuscitated after the first three shocks, what would have been your priority?

If the patient is not successfully resuscitated after the first three defibrillations, the pulse should be assessed. If absent, CPR should be performed for 1 minute. It is important to evaluate the effectiveness of the CPR by assessing for a carotid pulse during chest compressions.

After 1 minute of CPR has been performed, reanalyzing the cardiac rhythm is indicated. If advised to do so by the AED, up to three more shocks should be delivered.

8. What are your priorities of management now that you have successfully restored the patient's pulse?

At this point, you must ensure that the patient's airway remains patent and that he receives the appropriate oxygenation therapy (BVM [Bag-Valve Mask] or NRB [Non-Rebreather Mask]). In the event that the patient's breathing returns but he remains unconscious, placing him in the recovery position and continually monitoring his pulse and respirations are the appropriate actions. Suction must be readily available in the event that the patient begins to vomit. In addition, the AED must remain attached to the patient should he go back into cardiac arrest.

After providing the appropriate postresuscitation management, the ALS ambulance arrives and takes over the care of the patient. He is rapidly transported to the closest appropriate facility with advanced interventions performed en route. You send your partner with the ALS unit to assist as needed.

9. Would your management have changed had this been a 6-year-old child?

Significantly. First of all, the adult AED is not recommended for use in patients less than 8 years of age or less than 25 kg (55 lbs). Pediatric or combination adult/pediatric AEDs are available. Children who go into cardiac arrest most commonly do so as a result of respiratory failure; therefore, early and aggressive airway support as well as effective CPR would be the most important management. Early notification of ALS support would still be an important factor to consider.

10. Are there any contraindications to the use of the AED?

The only definite contraindication to defibrillation is in the patient less than 8 years old or less than 55 pounds. There are other circumstances where defibrillation isn't likely to be effective. Your protocols may not allow you to treat patients who have traumatic injuries or hypothermia. Traumatically induced cardiac arrest is usually caused by hypovolemia, in which case asystole is usually the presenting rhythm. Management for cardiac arrest secondary to trauma includes CPR, control of hemorrhage, and rapid transport to a trauma center. Unfortunately, traumatic cardiac arrest has a very high mortality rate.

PATIENT OUTCOME/PATHOPHYSIOLOGY

The patient was delivered to the emergency department with a pulse and spontaneous respirations. After a 6-day stay in the hospital, he was discharged to a local cardiac rehabilitation facility with no permanent disability.

Cardiopulmonary arrest in the adult is most often the result of myocardial infarction (heart attack), which produces a cardiac dysrhythmia, such as ventricular fibrillation. Ventricular fibrillation, which does not produce a pulse, is defined as a "quivering" of the myocardium due to a generalized, chaotic electrical discharge of cardiac cells. Normally, the electrical conduction system of the heart functions in an organized pattern, allowing for normal atrial and ventricular contraction. The single most important therapy for this cardiac disturbance is early defibrillation. The goal of defibrillation is to temporarily stop the heart from "fibrillating" so that normal electrical conduction can resume.

EVALUATION

1. The most common initial cardiac rhythm in cardiac arrest is:
   a. ventricular tachycardia
   b. ventricular fibrillation
   c. pulseless electrical activity
   d. asystole

2. The most important initial management for the patient in witnessed cardiac arrest is:
   a. to perform 1 minute of CPR
   b. to call for an ALS ambulance
   c. to assess the need for defibrillation
   d. to immediately transport the patient to the hospital

3. You have just performed the initial defibrillation with an AED on a 45-year-old patient in cardiac arrest. What should happen next?
   a. you should check for the presence of a pulse
   b. CPR should be performed for 1 to 2 minutes
   c. the patient should be transported at once
   d. the patient's cardiac rhythm should be reanalyzed

4. The AED is designed to deliver the initial defibrillation at how many joules?
   a. 50
   b. 100
   c. 200
   d. 300

5. Defibrillation with an AED is not recommended in which of the following cases?
   a. if the patient has been in cardiac arrest for more than 5 minutes
   b. if the patient is over the age of 65 or over 200 pounds
   c. if the patient is under 8 years of age or under 55 pounds
   d. if the cardiac arrest was not witnessed and bystander CPR was not started

6. CPR has been in progress on a 60-year-old woman for approximately 10 minutes. Upon arrival at the scene, you should first:
   a. immediately defibrillate the patient
   b. notify the coroner as this patient is dead

c. confirm that the patient is in cardiac arrest

d. continue CPR for 1 minute prior to attaching the AED

7. Prior to defibrillating with an AED, the EMT's most important action is to:

a. confirm the absence of a pulse

b. ensure that patient contact has ceased

c. perform adequate CPR for 1 to 2 minutes

d. call for an ALS ambulance to respond to the scene

8. You have just performed the second defibrillation on a cardiac arrest patient. The AED advises you to check the patient. You should:

a. make sure that the pads are properly placed

b. assess the patient's level of consciousness

c. check for the presence of a carotid pulse

d. make sure that nobody is in contact with the patient

9. Which of the following statements is TRUE regarding the AED?

a. All AEDs have an autoanalyze function.

b. The AED will analyze accurately in the back of a moving ambulance.

c. After the initial shocks, subsequent shocks are delivered at 360 joules.

d. If the patient is moving, analysis of the rhythm will not occur.

10. You have successfully resuscitated a patient from cardiac arrest with an AED. After confirming the presence of a pulse, you should:

a. immediately transport the patient

b. place the patient in the recovery position

c. assess the adequacy of the patient's breathing

d. remove the AED to avoid accidental defibrillation

8

I Think He Is Dead

Objectives

At the conclusion of this scenario, the participant will be able to:

1. Describe the signs of obvious death.

2. Discuss when the defibrillator (AED) will advise to shock and when it will not.

3. Describe the three things that must be checked when a pulse returns after cardiac arrest.

SCENARIO

Your EMS unit is dispatched for a "man down" at 7775 W. Hartford Street. The dispatcher reports that a woman had checked on an elderly parent and found him on the bed; she reported "I think he's dead."

You respond to the scene with lights and siren. When you arrive you find a crying woman on the front porch. "I called him last night. He said he didn't feel well. I came over this morning and found him. . . . well, I think he may have died." You find out where the patient is and carefully make your way to him as you apply body substance isolation.

You find a male patient in his 70s lying face down in bed. You attempt to arouse the patient by shaking him and shouting. No response.

1. What facts have you gathered thus far to determine down time?

The woman stated that she last had contact with her father the night before. She also went into the house and found him lifeless, apparently dead. Unfortunately this does not tell us how long the patient was actually down. The obvious question is whether he was stricken last night after the phone call, a short time ago, or somewhere in between.

2. What are signs of obvious death that would cause you to not resuscitate the patient?

Most EMS systems have protocols that state when resuscitation isn't necessary. In some cases there are injuries that are too severe (e.g. brain matter showing) or the down time is too long for the patient to have any chance of survival. In these cases it is recognized that resuscitation is futile. These signs include rigor mortis (rigidity of the body after death), gross dependent lividity (pooling of the blood in low places that presents with a purple color in the skin), decomposition, or peeling of the skin.

3. What equipment should you have at the patient's side?

You should be prepared for a code (cardiac arrest). This includes a full first-in bag with BVM, oxygen, suction, and AED.

You examine the patient and find him pulseless and apneic. He does not have any signs of obvious death that indicate a prolonged down time. His skin temperature appears warm to the touch. You and your partner move him to the floor and immediately cut off his pajama top. Your partner provides CPR for the few moments it takes you to apply the AED electrodes. You and your partner clear the patient and press "analyze." The AED analyzes and advises a shock.

4. Why is the defibrillator advising a shock?

The AED will advise you to deliver a shock for only one reason: It detects a shockable rhythm. These rhythms include ventricular fibrillation and ventricular tachycardia. The AED does not check a pulse—only the cardiac rhythm.

You clear the patient and administer a shock. The AED analyzes and advises again to shock. Again the patient is cleared and a shock delivered. The AED analyzes once more. No shock is advised.

5. When will the defibrillator advise not to shock?

The defibrillator in this case would read "no shock advised" because the patient is no longer in a shockable rhythm. This could be good (the rhythm is a good, organized rhythm that may produce a pulse) or bad (the patient is in asystole or another bad and unshockable rhythm).

You check the patient's pulse and find it present. It is weak and a bit slow, but it is there.

6. What else must you assess and why?

There are three things that must be checked when a pulse returns after cardiac arrest. First you must check for breathing. If the breathing is inadequate or absent (as is often the case after cardiac arrest) ventilations will be required. Next, determine if the pulse is producing a blood pressure. Checking for a radial pulse gives some idea of perfusing to the extremities before a blood pressure (BP) reading can be taken. Finally, monitor the patient's pulse carefully. In some cases the patient will go back into cardiac arrest. This should be detected promptly for best chances of another successful defibrillation.

The patient begins turning his head slightly. You see some heaving motions in his chest as he tries to breathe. His chest is moving slightly at a rate of about 6 per minute.

7. What type of oxygen and/or ventilation would you provide for this patient? Why?

You provide assisted ventilations with a bag-valve mask that is connected by reservoir to oxygen.

You begin transport to the closest hospital. The patient is handed off to the ED with a pulse. He is lightly chewing on the oral airway but hasn't regained consciousness. As you hand over BVM ventilations to the waiting respiratory therapist you are congratulated for your work on this call.

PATIENT OUTCOME/PATHOPHYSIOLOGY

The patient was transferred to the intensive care unit (ICU), where he lived overnight but died the next day. A few days later you transport another patient to the hospital and speak to the physician who was on duty that day. She explains to you that even though you were able to get a pulse back the patient had experienced a significant anterior wall myocardial infarction. This involved the left ventricle—the largest and strongest and without which the patient couldn't survive. Despite medications that maintained his blood pressure, there was too much damage to the heart for the patient to survive.

The physician sees disappointment in your eyes. She explains, "You did all you could—and very well. It's not your fault. Some patients just can't be saved."

EVALUATION

1. Which is not a sign of obvious death?

   a. rigor mortis

   b. cardiac arrest

   c. dependent lividity

   d. decomposition

2. The presence of a carotid pulse and the absence of radial pulses in a patient whose pulse has returned after defibrillation indicates:

   a. aneurysm

   b. bilateral radial occlusion

   c. hypotension

   d. hypertension

3. Most patients who experience out-of-hospital cardiac arrest die.

   a. true

   b. false

4. A "no shock advised" message from an AED indicates the patient has a pulse.

   a. true

   b. false

5. Before pressing the "shock" button on an AED you should do all of the following EXCEPT:

   a. contact medical direction

   b. assure everyone has cleared the patient

   c. assure the patient is pulseless

   d. press the analyze button

6. Which of the following statements about a patient whose pulse has returned after defibrillation is false?

   a. The patient may or may not regain breathing.

   b. The patient won't go back into cardiac arrest.

   c. The patient is likely to have low blood pressure.

   d. The patient won't always regain a gag reflex.

7. Which cardiac rhythm won't be shocked by an automated defibrillator?

   a. V-Tach with a pulse

   b. V-Tach without a pulse

   c. asystole

   d. fine ventricular fibrillation

8. You are working EMS at a large gathering. You witness an elderly man go down not far from where your EMS vehicle is. You arrive to find him in cardiac arrest. You have your defibrillator, oxygen, and BVM at the patient's side. You should:

   a. apply the AED immediately

   b. use the oxygen and BVM immediately, then apply the AED

   c. contact medical direction

   d. first call ALS, then use the BVM with supplemental oxygen, then apply the AED

9. You are called to a scene where a terminal cancer patient has been found without breathing or pulse by family members. They called EMS. You arrive to find the patient in cardiac arrest without signs of a prolonged down time. The family wants you to "check him," but feels he should be left as is and not resuscitated due to his terminal condition. They have no documentation and no DNR order. You should:

   a. honor their wishes and verify that the patient has died

   b. check ABCs and call medical direction

   c. check ABCs, begin BLS (Basic Life Support) measures, and call medical direction

   d. check ABCs, call the patient's family physician, and begin BLS care if advised to

10. After analyzing, the AED could shock a patient with a pulse.

   a. true

   b. false

9

MY HEART IS SKIPPING BEATS

Objectives

At the conclusion of this scenario, the participant will be able to:

1. Discuss causes of irregular heartbeats.

2. Identify immediate actions necessary in a witnessed cardiac arrest.

3. List assessment priorities for patients with irregular heartbeats.

SCENARIO

Your ambulance has been dispatched to a retirement community. Dispatch reports that the caller, an elderly male, stated that his heart is skipping beats. Your estimated time of arrival is less than 5 minutes.

1. What are your thoughts regarding the caller's complaint?

When a patient reports that his heart is skipping beats you have many possible causes. The first thing to note, however, is that the patient is actually able to sense or feel his own heart beating. This is termed "palpitations." The average heart beats an estimated 115,000 times a day. Most of us go through an entire day without feeling the beating of our own heart. We usually only feel our heart beating after strenuous exertion due to an increase in blood pressure. The irregularity of the heart's rhythm is termed "dysrhythmia." It literally means an abnormal rhythm. The sense of skipping beats may be due to either "missed" beats or extra beats that are not normally present. Many patients have irregular heart rhythms. Most are due to electrolyte imbalance or chemicals ingested or inhaled by patients. For example, potassium or calcium derangements may lead to dysrhythmias. Other items that most people do not consider harmful may also lead to dysrhythmias, for example, nicotine from cigarettes and caffeine, just to name a few. Also be aware that dysrhythmias may be life threatening if they occur secondary to an acute cardiac event like AMI (Acute Myocardial Infarction) or CHF (Congestive Heart Failure).

2.   What actions will you take while en route to the scene?

You and your partner need to assign tasks such as who will perform the patient assessment, vital sign collection, oxygen administration, and so on. You will also need to gather your personal protective equipment, which should include gloves and eye protection at a minimum.

Upon arrival at the residence you ensure scene safety. You approach the home and knock on the door. You are invited in by an elderly male, approximately 60 years old, who states that he was the caller. You follow him to the living room where he sits down on the couch. After the patient gives his consent you begin your assessment.

3.   What type of consent must be secured before you can begin assessing and treating this patient?

Adult patients who are conscious, alert, and oriented must give "informed consent" before you can begin assessing and treating them. Informed consent requires you to explain that you are going to perform a physical exam and that based on your findings you will intervene accordingly. You will explain the therapies before you perform them. Remember that adult patients who are oriented have the right to refuse all or part of intended actions.

You begin your focused history and physical exam. You have already recognized that the patient is conscious and alert. His skin color is good and his respirations are deep and at an adequate rate. His pulse is present at the wrist and slightly irregular. You decide to begin questioning the patient about his complaint.

4.   What questions would be appropriate to ask regarding his complaint of a skipping heart?

You would begin by asking the patient to further describe his complaint. Begin with an open-ended question. You might continue by asking him if he presently feels like it is skipping beats. This might determine if the event has already passed or is ongoing. You should also inquire if there is any pain associated with the feeling. Does he feel short of breath or have nausea? Then try to establish a timeline as to when the symptom began and what he was doing when it started. Ask whether or not he has had similar episodes in the past and if so what the diagnosis was. Dysrhythmias may also cause a drop in blood pressure. You should also ask about whether the patient feels weak or faint.

The patient reports that the rhythm of his heart began feeling irregular about 30 minutes ago. He was cleaning the garage when it began. He came inside and rested for a while but it never improved. He denies pain or shortness of breath. He also denies feeling faint or weak. He states that this has never happened in his past. He denies any past medical problems at all.

5. What of the above information requires more in-depth questioning?

The patient stated that he was cleaning the garage when this began. You must inquire whether or not the patient may have been exposed to chemicals or other toxins. Ask if the patient was working with items such as fertilizer, pesticides, or abrasive chemicals. These types of chemicals can affect the nervous system of the body, including cardiac regularity.

The patient denies exposure to any toxins. He was just sweeping out the garage when it began. You direct your partner to perform vital signs as you begin your physical exam. Your primary survey reveals that the patient's ABCs are still present. He continues to deny pain or shortness of breath. His breath sounds are clear and equal bilaterally. His abdomen is soft to palpation with no pain or masses detected. His lower extremities are clear with no swelling. Pulses, sensation, and motor function are within normal limits. His upper extremities are also unremarkable with equal grip-strength noted. Palpation of his radial pulse allows you to feel his irregular pulse rate of 70/minute. You are unable to detect any pattern to his irregularity. Your partner reports the following vital signs: B/P 118/70, HR of 70/irregular, RR of 18, SpO$_2$ of 95 percent on room air. He also reports that the patient's pupils are equal, round, and reactive.

6. What would your next action be?

Following your focused history and physical exam you need to begin oxygen administration. One potential cause for heartbeat irregularity is an insufficient amount of available oxygen. The next step would be to begin oxygen administration, followed by preparation for transport.

You begin oxygen administration at 4 Lpm with a nasal cannula and move the patient to the stretcher. You continue to assess the patient by gathering a SAMPLE history. The patient denies any medication allergies or medication use. He reports no past medical problem. He last ate 2 hours ago.

7. What should you do after moving the patient to the ambulance?

You should reassess your interventions. Following the initiation of oxygen administration you should ascertain if the patient continues to have the irregular heartbeat. This should be done not only by asking the patient if symptoms continue but also by palpating his radial pulse again.

You place the patient in the back of the ambulance and begin nonemergency transport to the patient's hospital of choice some 10 minutes away. You continue to administer oxygen and you reassess his vital signs. Suddenly the patient states that he doesn't feel well. You see panic and apprehension on his face. He suddenly clutches his chest and his eyes roll, looking up and back.

8. What action would you now perform?

Reassess. This is a sudden change requiring potential intervention. Begin by repeating your assessment of airway, breathing, and circulation.

You reassess the patient and determine that he is not breathing and he has no pulse. You immediately prepare a bag-valve mask for ventilation. You insert an oral airway and administer two breaths. You direct your partner (driver) to detour to the closest hospital.

You immediately apply an AED device. The machine advises a shock. You push the shock button. It reassesses. It advises a second shock. You again push the shock button. It is repeated for the third time.

9. What follows this third shock?

   You perform another pulse check. Standard sequences of care when utilizing an AED call for three shocks followed by a pulse check and then CPR if necessary.

   Following the third shock the patient begins to cough and gag himself on the oral airway. You are able to palpate a carotid pulse.

10. What should be done with the oral airway?

    The oral airway must be removed. Following the third shock the circulatory system of the patient has been restored. The patient is now breathing and gagging on the oral airway. If it is not removed the patient may vomit and then aspirate material into his lungs.

    You find that the patient is now awake and somewhat dazed as to what has just happened. He is breathing adequately and complains of a burning sensation as he points to the AED pads. You place the patient back on oxygen but this time at 15 Lpm with a nonrebreather mask. You continue your reassessment and have just completed performing another set of vital signs as you arrive at the emergency department. You deliver the patient to the emergency room (ER) staff, where you give your report to the physician and nursing personnel. You leave the ER and prepare for the next call.

PATIENT OUTCOME/PATHOPHYSIOLOGY

The patient was assessed by emergency department personnel. A 12-lead EKG revealed that the patient was suffering from multiple premature ventricular contractions (PVCs). This is a condition that can disrupt the organized electrical activity of the heart. It is suspected that the patient had one of these PVCs occur during a vulnerable period of a heart contraction. This is known to cause the heart to stop in some patients. The patient has been hospitalized and will undergo numerous exams to determine the cause of these PVCs. One exam will actually "map" the electrical pathways of the heart to see if it can determine the area causing these abnormal beats.

EVALUATION

1. What term is utilized to describe the patient's ability to sense an irregular heart rhythm?
   a. dysrhythmia
   b. angina
   c. flutter sensation
   d. palpitation

2. Which of the following chemicals could cause an irregular heart rhythm?
   a. Windex
   b. cat litter
   c. pesticides
   d. Armor-all

3. Which of the following would you want to provide early in the care of this patient?
   a. epi-pen
   b. nitroglycerin
   c. oxygen
   d. syrup of ipecac

4. What is the first thing you would do when there is a change in the patient's condition?
   a. initiate oxygen at 15 Lpm with a nonrebreather mask
   b. reassess LOC (Loss/Level of Consciousness), airway, breathing, and circulation
   c. begin ventilation with a BVM device
   d. initiate chest compressions

5. Oral airways are sized by using which two anatomical landmarks?
   a. tip of the nose to the lower tip of the ear lobe
   b. angle of the jaw and corner of the mouth
   c. lips to adam's apple
   d. utilize the same sizing technique as a nasal-pharyngeal airway

6. Oral airways are indicated for which of the following patients?
   a. unconscious patient
   b. semiconscious patient
   c. unconscious patient with no gag reflex
   d. none of the above

7. It is acceptable to continue chest compressions and BVM ventilations during a shock delivered by an AED.
   a. true
   b. false

8. Which of the following could lead to an irregular heart rhythm?
   a. nicotine
   b. decaffeinated coffee
   c. nitro patches
   d. white-out

9. If the patient had been exposed to chemicals in the garage, who should be notified?

   a. a second EMS unit

   b. law enforcement personnel

   c. fire department hazardous materials team

   d. all of the above

10. If, following your assessment, you determine chemical exposure, who needs to be decontaminated?

   a. the patient

   b. you and your partner

   c. all of your equipment

   d. all of the above

10

I HAVE PAIN
IN MY CHEST

Objectives

At the conclusion of this scenario, the participant will be able to:

1. List treatment priorities for acute angina.

2. Describe situations in which patients should take their own nitroglycerin.

3. Identify indications that treatment has been effective.

SCENARIO

You and your partner are providing "stand-by" coverage at a large air-show event. Yours is one of five mobile teams providing coverage for some 5,000 spectators. You are covering your sector while riding in your medical golf cart. Someone waves you down and directs you to an elderly man sitting on a barricade clutching his chest.

1. What is your primary concern in this situation?

   Elderly patients who are found clutching their chest may be suffering from several complaints ranging from shortness of breath to cardiac-related chest pain. You are aware that cardiac chest pain may quickly lead to cardiac arrest.

   As you approach the man you are able to see that he looks pale and has beads of sweat on his face and neck. He appears very anxious.

2. What are your thoughts concerning this quick visual assessment?

   Patients who have cardiac-related pain, which may be indicative of myocardial infarction, often-times present with altered color and skin perfusion. This patient is pale and has evidence of diaphoresis. This patient will fit into an emergent category. This would require a short scene time.

You approach the patient and introduce yourself. He states that he has been having severe chest pain for about 5 minutes. He says that the pain is dull, located in the center of his chest, and he can feel it travel to his neck. He sat down hoping that it would go away but it hasn't. He is also looking for his wife because she has his medicine in her purse.

3. With this information, what are your primary considerations as to the cause?

   Chest pain may have many causes. This patient complains of dull chest pain, which radiates into his neck. It has not been relieved by rest. This in conjunction with his pale color and diaphoresis must raise suspicion of a cardiac cause. The two most common causes of cardiac-related pain are angina pectoris and acute myocardial infarction. Angina is caused when a portion of the heart is lacking sufficient oxygen to meet its demand. The cause is usually a spasm of a coronary vessel or a partial blockage of a coronary vessel as the result of coronary artery diseases such as arteriosclerosis or atherosclerosis. It is oftentimes relieved by rest, oxygen, and/or nitroglycerin administration. Acute myocardial infarction (AMI) is also known as a heart attack. It results when a coronary artery becomes occluded by a clot or thrombus. The pain of an AMI is not relieved by rest, oxygen, or nitroglycerin. It is a true emergency that may cause serious damage to the heart if not corrected.

You obtain permission to treat. You sit the patient on your transport vehicle. You direct your partner to initiate oxygen therapy at 15 Lpm with a nonrebreather mask. You begin your focused history and physical exam. You note that the patient is awake, alert, and oriented. His airway is open and remains patent. A palpable radial pulse is present at 96/minute. His skin remains diaphoretic. You ask the patient to describe the pain and then rate it on a 1–10 scale.

4. What are common descriptions that patients may utilize when describing cardiac-related chest pain?

   Patients often describe cardiac-related chest pain as being dull or heavy in nature. Phrases such as "I feel like I have an elephant sitting on my chest" or "I feel like I have a vice around my chest" are often utilized. Remember that patients do not have true pain-sensing nerves on their hearts. Instead, reports of pain are sent to the brain by utilizing other pain-sensing pathways. Also, remember that a patient's description of pain is personal and may not follow "typical" responses. Patients with sharp chest pain may be experiencing a heart attack just the same as someone with a dull, heavy, weighted chest pain.

5. Why do you ask the patient to grade the pain utilizing a 1–10 scale?

   By asking the patient to grade his pain on a 1–10 scale (10 being the worst pain he has ever experienced and 0 being no pain at all) it allows the medical provider to determine the patient's sense of pain intensity. Also, by frequent repeat assessments it allows us to determine if the pain has improved or worsened.

You ask your partner to perform a check of vital signs as you begin your physical exam. You note that the patient seems less anxious now that you are caring for him and providing oxygen administration. The patient is still diaphoretic. Auscultation of the chest reveals present and clear bilateral lung sounds. The abdomen is soft with no complaints of nausea. No palpable abdominal masses are noted. The extremities are normal except for diaphoresis of the upper arms.

6. Why is it important to listen to breath sounds when the patient is complaining of cardiac-related chest pain?

Although the symptoms reported cause a high index of suspicion of a cardiac-related cause, we cannot rule out other situations that would cause similar complaints. One such situation that may cause chest pain and shortness of breath is a spontaneous pneumothorax. Spontaneous pneumothorax occurs when a weakened portion of a lung gives way, allowing air to become trapped between the lung and the rib cage. This oftentimes occurs during exertion, such as walking at an air show. We are able to rule out this potential cause by auscultation of breath sounds. Present bilateral breath sounds indicate that the lungs are expanding normally.

Your partner reports the following vital signs: B/P 150/82, HR 96, RR 20, and an SpO₂ reading of 99 percent on oxygen. Pupils are also equal, round, and reactive to light. You are just about to begin transport to an awaiting ambulance when the patient's wife arrives. She immediately rushes to her husband's side and asks what is wrong. He tells her of his chest pain and asks if she still has his nitroglycerin tablets in her purse. She states that she does as she retrieves them from her bag. You radio your incident command that you will be bringing a patient to the ambulance staging area momentarily.

7. What is nitroglycerin and why would this patient have this medication?

Nitroglycerin (Nitrostat) is a medication that causes vasodilation of coronary and peripheral vessels. When administered to a patient with an acute coronary syndrome it reduces the workload of the heart and may allow the vessels to dilate or open enough to improve blood flow to the heart that is lacking oxygen.

More than likely this patient has had a prior coronary event such as angina pectoris or even a previous AMI and has been prescribed this medication by a doctor in the event of another recurrence.

You continue to gather your SAMPLE history as your partner begins driving you to the awaiting ambulance. The patient's wife is also on the medical cart. The patient explains that he began having this chest pain while walking. He was walking faster than usual because there was so much to see. As soon as the pain began he sat down but it never improved. He admits to a shellfish allergy. The only medication that he takes is Coreg and a daily aspirin. This is in conjunction with his nitroglycerin tablets, which he only takes if he has chest pain. His past medical history includes an AMI some 8 years ago, which was treated with a clot-buster drug. He last ate several hours ago.

8. What is Coreg and why would he take an aspirin every day?

Coreg (aka Carvedilol) is a medication that fits into a class of drugs called "beta blockers." When this medication is given to patients it prevents the heart from speeding up too quickly or too rapidly. It also restricts the force of each contraction. This is beneficial for some cardiac patients because it forces the heart to remain in a "nonexcited" state. This has been shown to reduce the incident of sudden cardiac death in patients following AMI recovery.

Aspirin is often prescribed to patients at risk for cardiac complications or those who have already suffered a cardiac event. It decreases the likelihood of heart attack.

Your patient informs you that his doctor told him to take the nitroglycerin tablets whenever anything like this occurs. You are aware that your medical director's standing orders allow you to assist in the administration of this medication if needed. He withdraws and takes one very small tablet and places it under his tongue. Within seconds he begins to complain of a headache, which he says is normal. Two or 3 minutes after taking the medication he says his pain is gone. He rates it as a 0 on a 1–10 scale.

9. Why did the patient suffer a headache following nitroglycerin administration?

Nitroglycerin causes dilation of coronary as well as peripheral vessels. After taking this medication the patient's cerebral vessels also began to dilate. This oftentimes causes a headache as the brain vessels increase in size. This is usually a transient complaint of those taking nitroglycerin.

You arrive at the ambulance staging area. The patient agrees to go to the hospital with the ambulance personnel to be checked out. You give your report to your fellow EMS personnel who will provide transport. After completing a brief contact form you and your partner return to your designated sector to continue your duty.

PATIENT OUTCOME/PATHOPHYSIOLOGY

Your patient was transported to the hospital by fellow EMS personnel. There he was diagnosed with a condition called exertional chest pain related to angina pectoris. He was hospitalized for follow-up. Cardiac catheterization the following day revealed that he had multiple vessel disease, which would require bypass surgery. Even though he did not have a heart attack, this chest pain event may have saved his life.

EVALUATION

1. Acute anginal chest pain or "exertional chest pain" is usually relieved by which of the following?
   a. rest
   b. oxygen
   c. nitroglycerin
   d. all of the above

2. Exertional chest pain is caused by:
   a. a thrombus blocking a coronary vessel
   b. plaque that obstructs a coronary artery
   c. inadequate blood delivery to the heart during times of increased need
   d. none of the above

3. Nitroglycerin has which of the following actions?
   a. vessel constrictor
   b. vessel dilator
   c. heart pain medication
   d. increases oxygen transport

4. Cardiac chest pain may be described as which of the following?

   a. sharp chest pain
   b. dull chest pain
   c. pain that radiates to the arm or neck
   d. all of the above

5. Patients who are complaining of chest pain should have an AED applied.

   a. true
   b. false

6. How should you have patients relate the severity of cardiac-related chest pain?

   a. in their own words
   b. with terms such as *very severe, severe, less severe,* or *not present*
   c. utilize a 1–10 scale
   d. DeBakey pain scale

7. One expected side effect of nitroglycerin is which of the following?

   a. worsening of pain initially followed by improvement
   b. nausea
   c. change in vision
   d. headache

8. One potential side effect of nitroglycerin is which of the following?

   a. increase in blood pressure
   b. decrease in blood pressure
   c. increase in heart rate
   d. decrease in heart rate

9. What effects can a daily aspirin cause?

   1. decreased rate of blood clotting
   2. increased rate of blood clotting
   3. thinning of the blood
   4. thickening of the blood

   a. 1 and 3
   b. 2 and 4
   c. 1, 2, and 4
   d. 2, 3, and 4

10. How should nitroglycerin tablets be administered?

   a. the patient should swallow the tablet
   b. the patient should chew the tablet but not swallow
   c. the patient should allow the tablet to dissolve under the tongue
   d. any of the above is acceptable

11

POSSIBLE STROKE

Objectives

At the conclusion of this scenario, the participant will be able to:

1. Recognize the signs and symptoms of acute CVA (stroke).

2. Describe the assessment of the patient with a suspected CVA.

3. List the principles of management for the patient with a CVA.

SCENARIO

A call is received at 1705 from a local assisted-living center for a 78-year-old woman with a possible stroke. The dispatcher attempted but was unable to obtain additional information. Your response time to the scene is approximately 6 minutes.

1. Any special considerations or thoughts while responding to the scene?

    Due to the lack of information regarding the status of the patient (i.e., conscious or not), while en route, you should have the dispatcher recontact the facility and attempt to gather more patient information. With such little initial information, the EMT should prepare for the absolute worst, such as cardiopulmonary arrest. It is much easier to simply set the AED aside if you do not need it as opposed to having to make a mad dash to the ambulance to retrieve it. Also, the time of call (1705) puts you right in the middle of rush-hour traffic. The driver must ensure that due regard is paid to the other motorists and pedestrians around him.

    You arrive on the scene at 1711 and are escorted to a room where you find an elderly female sitting in a chair. You note that she has a marked left-side facial droop and her left arm is lying flaccid on the bed beside her. She does not appear to be in any obvious distress.

2. What information have you gathered during your general impression of this patient?

Your general impression should be that of a conscious patient who does not appear to be injured. Her initial presentation appears to be that of a stroke; however, the specifics of her presentation, such as time of onset and whether or not these signs are new or reflective of a previous stroke, must be established.

As you approach the patient, you introduce yourself to her and ask her how she is doing. She looks up at you with a fearful look in her eyes and then glances at her left arm. The nurse states that they attempted to communicate with the patient, but she would not talk to them.

During your initial assessment, you note that her airway is open and patent, her respirations are 18 with good air movement, and her heart rate is 66 and strong. You quickly scan her entire body and do not see any obvious signs of trauma.

3. What is the significance, if any, of the patient not talking to you?

First of all, the look of fear in the patient's eyes and the fact that she is not talking does not reflect an unwillingness to speak, but rather an inability to speak. This is called expressive aphasia and is a common finding in stroke patients.

4. How are you going to communicate with this patient?

Just because the patient cannot speak does not mean that she cannot understand. In talking to her, you should attempt to establish a means of communication specific to her needs, such as nodding her head to your yes or no questions or, if she is able to, writing her responses to your questions with her unaffected hand. If these strategies are not possible, you will have to rely on the staff to answer any questions.

5. What other questions might you ask the staff regarding this patient?

Because she was found sitting in a chair, you must ascertain whether or not she fell and was placed in the chair by the staff. Though your visual exam during the initial assessment did not reveal any obvious trauma, you must still rule this out. Additionally, you should inquire about the patient's past medical history, specifically asking about conditions that would put her at high risk for a stroke such as hypertension, diabetes, or cardiac problems. In addition, a list of her current medications should be obtained.

You find it very difficult to communicate with the patient using various strategies. As your partner applies a nonrebreather mask to the patient, the staff member that is responsible for the patient's daily activities tells you that the patient was "fine" 30–45 minutes prior. When she came in to check on the patient, she was found in the chair, where she was previously left, in her present state.

After applying oxygen to the patient, your partner obtains a set of baseline vital signs. Her B/P is 160/90, pulse is 72, and her respirations are 18. The nurse presents a list of medications to you, which includes Vasotec and various vitamin supplements. She states that the patient has high blood pressure and has had several TIAs (transient ischemic attacks) over the past few weeks.

6. What have you learned from the information presented to you by the staff as well as her vital signs, past medical history, and medications?

Because the patient was last seen in a chair prior to the episode and then found in the same chair after the onset of symptoms, you can likely rule out trauma. Also, the events of this episode came within a short period of time. This is significant because if the patient is having a stroke, delivery to the appropriate facility within 3 hours after the onset of symptoms will potentially make her a candidate for medications that could halt the stroke process and minimize any permanent disability.

With regards to her blood pressure, 160/90 is not dangerously high, but high enough to warrant concern. The medication Vasotec is a frequently prescribed antihypertensive medication. Her history of hypertension confirms this. The history of recent TIAs should increase your index of suspicion. A transient ischemic attack, also called a small stroke, is an indicator that a "full-blown" stroke is likely to occur. The pathophysiology of the TIA and the cerebrovascular accident (CVA) will be discussed at the end of this case study.

7. How will this information affect your management of the patient?

The information provided to you will not have an affect on the management of the patient; however, the patient's condition will have a significant impact on your management. You are already providing the appropriate management for this patient (monitoring ABCs, 100 percent oxygen, etc.), but must be able to "switch gears" should the patient's condition take a turn for the worse. The information that has been provided to you will be of immense help to the emergency department staff in the definitive management of the patient.

You and your partner place the patient on the stretcher, position her in a semi-fowler position and begin transport to the hospital, which is approximately 7 miles away. Her condition remains unchanged throughout transport.

8. Are there any special considerations that you must be aware of during transport?

You must constantly ensure that the patient remains aware of her surroundings to include where she is at and where you are taking her. The loss of one's ability to communicate is a horrifying event. Make sure that you remain in a position where the patient can constantly see you and explain all procedures, if any, that you intend to perform. Because many stroke patients lose their gag reflex, you should constantly manage the airway and provide suction as needed. In addition, due to the tendency of the stroke patient to suddenly deteriorate, the EMT must be prepared to assist ventilations or perform CPR (have the AED ready).

You deliver the patient to the emergency department staff without incident. As you are moving the patient to the hospital stretcher, she looks at you with great appreciation. You smile at her, give your report to the nurse, and return to service.

After a detailed assessment in the emergency department as well as other diagnostic procedures, the patient was diagnosed with an acute ischemic stroke. After a 2-week stay in the hospital, she was returned to the assisted-living center with moderate neurologic deficit, which will be managed with rehabilitation.

A stroke, also called a cerebrovascular accident (CVA), occurs when a portion of the brain is deprived of oxygenated blood, resulting in necrosis (tissue death). There are two main types of strokes: the ischemic stroke (75 percent of all strokes) and the hemorrhagic stroke. The hemorrhagic stroke occurs due to the rupture of a cerebral blood vessel (an aneurysm), which not only causes injury to the area(s) of the brain beyond the rupture, but bleeding within the brain and increased intracranial pressure as well. The ischemic stroke occurs as the result of an occlusion (thrombus formation) in a cerebral artery with progressive arterial narrowing until oxygen beyond the area(s) of blockage is cut off altogether.

The patient in this case study was suffering from an ischemic stroke, which typically presents as a sudden inability to move one side of the body (hemiplegia) or weakness to one side of the body (hemiparesis). Other signs of an acute ischemic stroke include slurred speech, mental status changes, and pupillary changes. Remember that the left side of the brain controls the right side of the body and vice versa, so a patient that presents with weakness or paralysis to one side of the body is likely to be suffering from a stroke to the opposite side of the brain. The pupils, however, will be affected on the same side as the stroke. A transient ischemic attack (TIA) occurs due to a significant narrowing (but not total blockage) of a cerebral blood vessel resulting in ischemia beyond the area of narrowing. A TIA is a major warning sign that a full-blown stroke will soon occur. The signs and symptoms of a TIA are similar, if not identical, to that of a stroke; however, they tend to resolve within 24 hours.

EVALUATION

1. Which of the following statements regarding a CVA is true?
   a. Signs of a major stroke tend to present over a period of days.
   b. Paralysis to the left side of the body could indicate a left-sided stroke.
   c. Weakness to the right side of the body could indicate a left-sided stroke.
   d. Signs of a stroke are usually self-limited and resolve within 24 hours.

2. A patient presents with mental confusion, the inability to move the left side of his body, and a left-side facial droop. He should be assumed to be having:
   a. a right-sided stroke
   b. a right-sided TIA

c. a left-sided stroke

d. a left-sided TIA

3. Initial management for the patient suspected of suffering from a stroke includes:

   a. obtaining vital signs

   b. conducting a detailed physical exam

   c. assessing neurological signs

   d. assuring a patent airway

4. A patient suspected of having suffered a stroke is unable to talk. In managing this patient, the EMT should:

   a. assume that the patient cannot understand either

   b. increase his or her voice so the patient can hear

   c. talk to the patient as though he can understand

   d. focus his or her questions to a bystander or the patient's caregiver

5. A patient that is suffering from a stroke should be positioned:

   a. in a lateral recumbent position

   b. in a semi-sitting position

   c. in the prone position

   d. on the opposite side of the stroke

6. You discover a patient lying on the floor with the classic signs and symptoms of a stroke. In managing this patient, the EMT should:

   a. consider the possibility of trauma

   b. open the airway with the head-tilt

   c. apply a nasal cannula to the patient

   d. immediately place the patient in a seated position

7. The most reliable way for the EMT to determine whether or not a patient who presents with signs of a stroke is having an acute problem or manifesting signs of an old stroke is to:

   a. take the patient's vital signs

   b. obtain a thorough history

   c. observe the patient's response to oxygen

   d. perform a detailed physical exam

8. Risk factors for a stroke include which of the following?

   a. hypotension

   b. psychiatric problems

   c. high blood pressure

   d. chronic bradycardia

9. A stroke is the result of a blockage or rupture of a:

   a. coronary artery

   b. cerebral vein

   c. coronary vein

   d. cerebral artery

10. Permanent disability can be minimized if the patient suffering from a stroke is delivered to the emergency department within how many hours after the onset of symptoms?

    a. 3

    b. 6

    c. 9

    d. 12

12

MAN DOWN

Objectives

At the conclusion of this scenario, the participant will be able to:

1. Describe the appropriate assessment of patients suffering from medical illnesses and trauma events.

2. List causes of syncopal or near-syncopal episodes.

3. Discuss the appropriate treatment of patients recovering from a syncopal episode.

SCENARIO

EMS has been dispatched to a residence. The caller reported that her husband was unconscious, lying on the bathroom floor. At the time of her call she did not know if her husband was breathing or not.

1. What are your thoughts about this dispatch information?

   There is a high likelihood that this patient may be in cardiac arrest. The caller reported that the patient was unconscious but could not report whether the patient was breathing or not. Assume the worst.

2. What will you do while en route to the call?

   You and your partner need to determine who will be responsible for different tasks. As always, gather your personal protective equipment, including gloves and eye protection at a minimum. Unconscious patients, especially those in possible cardiac arrest, will require more than two EMS personnel if possible. Request assistance if available. Once you arrive on scene you need to ensure that the appropriate equipment is taken to the patient's side. Your first-in bag should include devices necessary to ventilate the patient along with an oxygen source. An AED should also be carried in. A long spine board would be helpful in transporting the patient as well as providing an appropriate CPR surface. Other spinal-motion-restriction equipment should also be taken to the patient in the event there was an unreported trauma.

You request that another EMS unit or supervisor respond to your assistance since cardiac arrest cannot be ruled out. Once you arrive on scene, and ensure that it is safe for you to enter, you and your partner carry all appropriate equipment into the home. There you are directed into the bathroom where you find a male patient, approximately 55 years old, leaning against the vanity. He has shaving cream on parts of his face and clothing. He is conscious and oriented to your questions. You see that he is holding a washcloth to his forehead. A small amount of blood is noted on the washcloth. He stated that he must have struck his head when he fell.

3. What would your next consideration be regarding this scenario?

    After you receive informed consent to treat you need to begin manual stabilization of the cervical spine. It is apparent that the victim fell to the floor with sufficient force to lacerate the soft tissues of the forehead. Spinal motion restriction is a consideration at this point.

After you secure informed consent to treat, you direct your partner to begin manual stabilization of the cervical spine. You inform the patient as to why this is necessary and he agrees. You also notify dispatch, by hand-held radio, that other responding units can be disregarded. You begin your assessment of the patient's chief complaint. He states that he was just getting ready to go to work. He was in the process of shaving when he says he just "blacked out."

4. What causes can you identify that would lead to someone "blacking out?"

    There are numerous causes that can be identified. First, let's define "blacking out." Blacking out usually means that the patient had a sudden onset of loss of consciousness or an onset of sudden loss of orientation. Some patients do not completely lose consciousness; however, they are so dazed that they lose perspective as to who they are, where they are at, and what is going on. Most laypersons use the term "fainting." In medicine this is called syncope. Syncope may have several causes. These include simple fainting, cardiac causes, a sudden change in position, standing for a prolonged time, and others. If the patient is tired or hasn't eaten, syncope is more likely.

Since your contact you have already determined that the patient is conscious, has a patent airway, is breathing, and has a radial pulse within normal limits. You continue with your focused history and physical exam. As you have already noted this patient is both a medical patient with concomitant trauma as well. You quickly perform a trauma assessment. You inquire as to whether the patient has any pain. He denies pain except for where the laceration is located on the right side of his forehead. You note a laceration that is approximately 1 inch in length and there is no active bleeding. Pupils are equal round and reactive. He denies neck pain and palpation is unremarkable.

5. What should your next step be?

   Following palpation of the patient's neck you need to apply an appropriately sized cervical collar. This, however, does not free your partner's responsibility to maintain manual stabilization. Manual stabilization will not be released until the patient is secured to a long spine board with appropriate cervical-motion-restriction devices secured.

   Following your intervention you continue your assessment. The patient denies chest pain or shortness of breath. Bilateral breath sounds are clear to auscultation. His abdomen is soft with no complaints of pain or nausea. Assessment of the patient's extremities is unremarkable. He has excellent motor/sensory function and pulses are palpable. The patient's back is unremarkable. You place the victim onto a long spine board and begin to secure him to the device. Once your partner is free you ask him to begin oxygen therapy, assess vital signs, and bandage the forehead laceration as you continue your assessment.

6. Which part of the focused history and physical exam should be performed next?

   Since you have completed your trauma assessment you should begin gathering a SAMPLE history. Hands-on assessment is generally more pertinent to the trauma patient, whereas information gained in a history is most pertinent to medical problems.

   Your partner reports the following vital signs: B/P 122/70, HR 88, RR 16, and a room air SpO$_2$ of 97 percent. The patient denied any complaints prior to blacking out. He states that he felt fine up until that time. He had just raised his head to begin shaving his mid-neck area. He denies any allergies or medication use other than occasional Tylenol. He has no past medical history. The patient states that he had not eaten breakfast as of yet. His only recollection of the event is that he was shaving and then he awoke on the floor.

   You and your partner move the patient, on the long spine board, from the bathroom to your awaiting stretcher. After your safety belts are applied you transfer the patient to your ambulance. You begin nonemergent transport to the patient's hospital of choice.

7. What actions will you perform during transport to the hospital?

   Continue oxygen administration throughout transport. You will need to reassess the patient and repeat vital signs. Also, check the bandage applied to the forehead laceration to ensure that there is no active bleeding. Be prepared to manage shock. Keep the patient at a normal temperature throughout transport. Radio the hospital with a patient report and your ETA.

   You continuously monitor and reassess your patient during transport. His reassessment remains unchanged and his vital signs are also normal. The patient has no further syncopal or near-syncopal episodes en route. You deliver the patient to the emergency department without incident. Following your verbal report you complete your run form and then return to service.

PATIENT OUTCOME/PATHOPHYSIOLOGY

The patient undergoes numerous exams in the emergency department. The physician believes that the patient suffered a syncopal episode due to a vaso-vagal response. Plainly put, the doctor believes that while the patient was shaving he applied pressure to the "pressure receptors" in his neck. This caused a sudden decrease in blood pressure that led to an inadequate supply of blood flow to the brain. This caused an immediate loss of consciousness leading to the patient's fall. Once the patient fell to the floor his blood pressure returned to normal and he regained consciousness. His spine was cleared by physician assessment. Sutures were placed to close the open laceration. The patient was discharged home with instructions to shave very carefully in the future.

Remember that syncope is a transient (or brief) loss of consciousness. The patient recovers quickly and without intervention. If the patient remains unconscious or retains an altered mental status for any amount of time it is not syncope. Things like diabetic conditions and stroke mimic syncope but are not classified as such.

EVALUATION

1. What is your first priority when responding to an unconscious patient?
   a. ensure an open airway
   b. determine level of consciousness
   c. ensure scene safety
   d. apply an AED

2. When assessing the victim of a fall, what should you assume?
   a. the patient will be treated under implied consent
   b. the victim may have a cervical spine injury
   c. the patient may have been drinking alcohol
   d. the patient has a closed head injury

3. What is the appropriate personal safety equipment that should be utilized with victims who have open lacerations?
   a. gloves and mask
   b. mask and goggles
   c. mask and impervious gowns
   d. gloves and protective eyeware

4. Which of the following are causes of syncopal episodes?
   a. diabetes
   b. stroke
   c. standing "at attention" for a prolonged time
   d. all of the above

5. When can manual stabilization of the neck be released in a suspected spinal injury?
   a. when the cervical collar has been applied
   b. when the victim is supine on the spine board

c. when the victim has been secured to the spine board with a cervical-motion-restriction device and straps

d. manual stabilization should be continued throughout transport

6. Which of the following generally provides the most information when treating a victim of a medical illness?

a. physical examination

b. vital signs

c. focused history

d. auscultation of breath sounds

7. Why is it important to assess the pupils of this patient?

a. required to be answered on the run form

b. may indicate whether or not this patient had a syncopal episode

c. may indicate presence of head injury

d. none of the above

8. It is not necessary to apply a cervical collar on a patient who denies neck pain.

a. true

b. false

9. Which of the following actions would be helpful if the patient's blood pressure was low?

a. administer small sips of water

b. elevate the patient's head

c. elevate the patient's legs

d. remove excess clothing

10. Pulse oximetry does which of the following?

a. determines whether or not the victim needs supplemental oxygen

b. represents the percentage of hemoglobin with oxygen bound to it

c. represents the percentage of normal hemoglobin circulating in the body

d. is helpful in assessing victims of carbon monoxide poisoning

13

My Son Had a Convulsion

Objectives

At the conclusion of this scenario, the participant will be able to:

1. Describe the assessment techniques for a pediatric patient.
2. List the signs and symptoms of a febrile seizure.
3. Define the management for the child suspected of having a febrile seizure.

SCENARIO

Dispatch notifies you of a frantic call from a mother who states that her 3-year-old son has had a convulsion. In and amongst the screaming of the mother, the dispatcher was able to hear a young child crying in the background. You and your partner depart for the scene at 1715.

1. From the dispatch information, what have you and your partner learned?

   Not much. You know that there is a frantic mother with a sick child. As for the child crying in the background, that does not mean that it is the patient. At this point, you don't even know if the patient is breathing or has a pulse.

   You arrive at the scene at 1721, where the mother, who is holding her child, meets you in the front yard. As you approach, the mother tells you that her son has been running a fever all day and is presently being treated for an ear infection. You notice that the conscious and crying child is wrapped in a water-soaked blanket and appears to be shivering. The mother tells you that her son was fine, then his "eyes rolled back into his head" and he began to shake all over. Evidently, this episode lasted approximately 2–3 minutes.

2. Based upon the general impression of the patient, are there any initial actions that you would or should take?

First of all, in order to avoid the "drawing of a crowd" you should bring the mother and child into the ambulance. Second, if this child indeed had a seizure as a result of fever, shivering is the body's way of producing heat and could cause an abrupt rise in body temperature, causing another seizure. Remove the blanket when you get in the ambulance.

As you begin your assessment of the child, you find that the 3-year-old is not very cooperative. He is clinging to mother and will not allow you to touch him. You notice that his skin is slightly red and you can see that he is obviously diaphoretic. His respirations are unlabored at a rate of 48. After a brief period of calming by the mother, you are able to obtain an apical pulse, which is 150 and strong.

3. What are your initial assessment findings? How do they correlate with the child's present condition?

Your initial assessment findings are essentially consistent with the child's complaint. The fact that the child is uncooperative is typical for a 3-year-old. His clinging to mom signifies that he recognizes her and this is a good indicator of the child's level of consciousness. Remember, when children no longer recognize their parents, they are in trouble. The skin color and quality are consistent with that of a "breaking fever." Respirations of 48, though slightly increased for this age group, are in all likelihood a manifestation of the fever. Tachycardia is also a classic manifestation of fever in children and adults alike.

4. What is an "apical" pulse and how is it obtained?

An apical pulse is obtained by placing the stethoscope directly over the child's heart, which is slightly to the left of the lower sternum, and counting the heart rate by auscultation.

As your partner hands the mother a pediatric face mask to hold near the child's face, she goes on to tell you that her son has no significant medical history other than the occasional "runny nose" and a few ear infections over the past year. He takes no medications regularly. She gave him pediatric Tylenol approximately 30 minutes ago. The child continues to cry and is resistant to the blow-by oxygen.

5. How should oxygen be delivered to a child who is uncooperative?

First of all, oxygen should be "offered" to a child. The EMT cannot assume that the child will be as rational as the adult in accepting the oxygen. In fact, upsetting a child who is already ill could cause an increase in the child's oxygen demand secondary to tachycardia and tachypnea, which in itself could have negative effects. Oxygen should be provided to a child based on the child's willingness to accept it, do not press the issue.

As you continue to work with the child, the mother takes the child's temperature. She has a relieved look on her face when she tells you that it is down to 100.3° from 104° earlier. By this time, your partner, who has children of his own, has managed to make the child smile by making a chicken's head out of a rubber glove.

6. Are there any other questions that you would ask the mother about this episode?

Yes, several. You should inquire about other signs and symptoms that could cause a fever. For example, questioning the mother about the presence of a stiff neck, which is indicative of meningitis, would be appropriate. Additionally, you should ask the mother if there is a possibility that her now "upwardly mobile" child could have gained access to the family medicine cabinet. Excessive aspirin ingestion can cause fever as well. Do not assume that this is just an ear-infection-related fever. Fever and seizures in children require a thorough assessment and history.

The mother asks you if transport to the hospital is necessary since the child's fever has obviously decreased significantly. You and your partner glance at each other as she asks you this. She further states that if possible, she would rather take the child to his pediatrician the next morning if he gets worse.

7. What is your response to the mother's request to transport via personally owned vehicle (POV)?

You should advise the mother that there are many causes of fever and seizures in children in addition to a simple ear infection, including meningitis, encephalitis, aspirin overdose, and sepsis. If the mother maintains her wish to take the child to the pediatrician, you should advise her of the consequences of refusing transport of her child, such as worsening of the fever, additional seizures, unconsciousness, and even death. Additionally, you should advise her to call 911 if the child gets worse and not to wait until the next morning. If she still maintains her stance, a signed refusal must be obtained.

After a brief period of deliberation, the mother agrees to allow you to transport the child to a local pediatric emergency department. You suggest that the mother bring a favorite toy of the child's to occupy him during transport. You notify the emergency department of your 5-minute arrival. Your transport is uneventful, as the child remains stable en route. You deliver the child to the emergency department and give a verbal report to the nurse.

PATIENT OUTCOME/PATHOPHYSIOLOGY

The patient was diagnosed in the emergency department with acute febrile seizure secondary to acute otitis media (middle ear infection). He was given more Tylenol (acetaminophen, a fever and pain reliever) and monitored for 2 hours prior to being discharged home.

Febrile seizures are among the most common pediatric calls that the EMT will respond to. A febrile seizure occurs secondary to an abrupt rise in body temperature. Note that it is not necessarily how high the temperature gets, but rather how quickly it gets there. The most common cause of the fever that leads to a seizure is an ear infection. Typically, the child will appear fine, then as his body temperature abruptly rises, the typical generalized motor (grand mal) seizure will occur, complete with the tonic-clonic extremity jerking. The seizure generally lasts less than 5 minutes and has ended by the time EMS arrives at the scene. It is important to point out that any infection that can cause a fever can result in a seizure, such as meningitis, encephalitis, aspirin overdose, and sepsis; therefore, all children with fever and seizures should be transported to the hospital for evaluation.

1. Febrile seizures in children are usually the result of which underlying problem?
   a. meningitis
   b. encephalitis
   c. ear infection
   d. severe sepsis

2. The most common type of seizure in the febrile child is the:
   a. petit mal
   b. grand mal
   c. tonic phase
   d. clonic phase

3. Which of the following statements regarding fever and seizures in children is true?
   a. The seizure generally lasts greater than 5 minutes.
   b. Most febrile seizures leave the child critically ill.
   c. All children with fever and seizures should be transported.
   d. Provided the fever has broke, the child is usually not transported.

4. The febrile seizure is caused by:
   a. cerebral hypoxia
   b. a temperature higher than 104°
   c. a temperature that rapidly falls
   d. an abrupt rise in body temperature

5. An ominous sign in an ill child includes:
   a. uncooperativeness
   b. being consoled only by a parent
   c. failure to recognize the parents
   d. uncontrolled crying and irritability

6. The medication most commonly given to children with fever is:
   a. Motrin
   b. Tylenol
   c. Aleve
   d. aspirin

7. What effect will shivering have on the body?
   a. it lowers body temperature
   b. it allows for muscular relaxation
   c. it produces body heat
   d. it is a mechanism to fight off infection

8. Signs of fever in a child include all of the following EXCEPT:
   a. bradycardia
   b. tachycardia
   c. tachypnea
   d. red skin color

9. Upon arrival at the scene of a child with an apparent febrile seizure, you note the child to be conscious and diaphoretic. Diaphoresis in a child following a febrile seizure generally indicates:
   a. an impending seizure
   b. a break in the fever
   c. severe hypovolemia
   d. increased heat production

10. You witness a child having a seizure. After the seizure ends, you should:
    a. rapidly cool the child
    b. evaluate the respirations
    c. establish an airway
    d. transport immediately

14

MY HUSBAND IS ACTING BIZARRELY

Objectives

At the conclusion of this scenario, the participant will be able to:

1. Explain the assessment process of the patient with diabetes.

2. Recognize the signs and symptoms of hypoglycemia.

3. List the indications, contraindications, and technique of administration for oral glucose.

SCENARIO

You and your partner receive a call to 1305 Mountain View Circle for a 35-year-old male who is acting "bizarre." The patient's wife made the call. The time is 1705 and your response time to the scene is approximately 7 minutes.

1. Are there any concerns or special considerations that you and your partner should discuss while en route to the scene?

   As with any call, scene safety is a top priority, especially when responding to a call such as this. A patient that is acting "bizarre" could imply a patient who is simply confused or one who is violently combative; therefore, law enforcement should make the scene safe prior to your entry. In addition, calling the dispatcher and attempting to obtain more information would be advisable.

   You arrive on scene at 1713 and note the presence of two sheriff's deputy's cars in the driveway. One of the deputies is standing on the front porch and motions for you to enter the residence. Upon entering the house, you see the patient, a young male who is talking to the other deputy. You notice that he has beads of sweat on his forehead and that his speech is slurred.

2. What is your general impression of this scene and the patient?

   Because law enforcement is at the scene and the deputy motions you inside, it is clear that the scene is safe for your crew to enter. The patient's general appearance and slurred speech could indicate a variety of problems. A more thorough assessment of this patient will be required to yield more information.

   Your initial assessment reveals a conscious patient with a patent airway. His respirations are slightly shallow at a rate of 24 and his heart rate is palpable at the radial site at a rate of 112 and weak. The remainder of the initial assessment is unremarkable. The patient's wife advises you that her husband is a diabetic. She returned home from work and found the patient in his present state. As you are talking to the patient, you do not note any strange odors on his breath.

3. Why specifically note the presence or absence of any strange breath odors?

   Due to the slurred speech of the patient, as well as a history of diabetes, you are evaluating specifically for the presence of a fruity odor on his breath. This could indicate a hyperglycemic state (diabetic coma). Do not be fooled if you smell what appears to be alcohol as this commonly mimics the acetone or fruity odor on the breath of a diabetic. Many times, diabetic patients are passed off as simply being "drunk" and are taken to jail, where they later die.

   Your partner applies oxygen with a nonrebreather mask; however, the patient will not allow this. He will tolerate a nasal cannula. As you begin to question the patient and his wife, your partner obtains a set of baseline vital signs. They are as follows: B/P 122/70, pulse 112, respirations 24 and slightly shallow.

4. What specific questions should be asked of the diabetic patient?

   In addition to the routine SAMPLE history that you should obtain on all patients, you should ask the following questions:

   - Do you take insulin? If so, when did you last take it and what was the dose?
   - Have you eaten today? If so, when and what was your last oral intake?
   - Have you been exerting yourself more than usual today?
   - Have you been ill at all recently?

   As you can tell from these questions, you are attempting to ascertain whether or not the patient's blood sugar could be high (failure to take his insulin, or taking too low of a dose), or whether it is low (he took too much insulin, took his regular dose but did not eat, has been exerting himself, vomiting meals, or experiencing illness, which may actually increase glucose needs; patients may actually reduce insulin during periods of illness when more may be necessary).

5. What is your next step in the management of this patient?

   Because this is a conscious medical patient, a focused history and physical exam are appropriate. The focused history should be based upon the questions regarding his diabetic history (see question 4). The physical exam should be pertinent to that of a diabetic such as blood glucose monitoring (if allowed by local protocol) as well as signs and symptoms suggestive of hypo/hyperglycemia.

The signs and symptoms of hypoglycemia and hyperglycemia are as follows:

Hypoglycemia (insulin shock)—

- Rapid onset
- Altered mental status
  - Ranging from mental confusion to combativeness to coma
- Diaphoresis
- Tachycardia and weak pulse

Hyperglycemia (diabetic coma)—

- Slow onset
- Altered mental status
  - In the later stages
- Warm, dry skin with poor skin turgor (dehydration)
- Tachycardia
- Excessive urination, hunger, or thirst
- Deep, rapid breathing (Kussmaul's respirations)
  - Acetone or fruity odor on the breath

The patient tells you that he is insulin dependent and that he remembers taking his insulin sometime this morning. He has been working all day trying to fix the transmission in his car and cannot remember when he last ate or checked his blood sugar. The wife brings his accu-check device, checks his blood sugar, and it reads 40.

6. What information that the patient provided you with, with the exception of the documented hypoglycemia, would lead you to suspect the same, even if you did not have an accu-check device?

There are several key points in what the patient has told you that should increase your index of suspicion for hypoglycemia. First, it was established that the patient took his insulin; how-ever, he has obviously been exerting himself all day and cannot remember when he last ate, which could lend to the assumption that he did not eat. Even in the absence of a documented blood sugar reading, it is clear that he has depleted his blood of sugar (glucose) in a number of ways including taking his insulin, which promotes the passage of sugar from the blood-stream and into the cell, as well as physical exertion, which utilizes significant amounts of sugar; and to make matters worse, he did not eat.

7. How should this patient be managed based upon these findings?

In addition to the oxygen that you are already providing, this patient needs sugar—whether it is a candy bar or the oral glucose from your ambulance. Oral glucose is a medication carried on a BLS unit that is clearly indicated in this situation. Because the patient is conscious and alert enough to swallow, he should be administered a tube of oral glucose, followed by a reassessment.

Prior to administering the glucose or any medication with the exception of oxygen, the EMT must contact medical control and obtain authorization. In some areas, locally established protocols may allow the EMT to administer oral glucose based upon standing orders. Once physician authorization has been obtained, the process of administering oral glucose is as follows:

- Remember the "five rights" of medication administration.
  - Right patient
  - Right medication
  - Right time
  - Right dose
  - Right route
- Check the medication to ensure that it is indeed oral glucose and that it is not expired.
- Place the oral glucose on a tongue depressor and rub it in between the patient's check and gum, where it can be absorbed by the mucous membrane. Alternatively, the patient may opt to simply squeeze the contents of the tube into his mouth himself.
  - Remember, oral glucose is a very thick, sticky substance, so pay attention to the patient's airway during administration in the event of inadvertent aspiration.
  - Have suction readily available should the patient begin to vomit.
  - NEVER administer oral glucose to patients if they are not conscious or not alert enough to swallow. Instead, consider requesting ALS and begin immediate transport with continual airway support.
  - Because it is often difficult for the EMT to determine whether or not the patient is suffering from hypoglycemia or hyperglycemia, if the patient is able to swallow, glucose should be administered.
- Assess the patient's response to the oral glucose.
- Notify medical control if the patient's condition remains unchanged. Additional glucose may need to be administered.

Following the appropriate management, the patient becomes more alert with fluent speech, his skin returns to its normal condition of pink, warm, and dry. The patient repeats an accu-check on himself and it now reads 88. His wife convinces him to be transported to the hospital for evaluation to make sure that nothing else is wrong and the patient consents. You transport the patient to a nearby hospital and deliver him to the emergency department staff in stable condition.

PATIENT OUTCOME/PATHOPHYSIOLOGY

The patient was diagnosed in the emergency department with acute hypoglycemia, most likely as the result of heavy exercise with no oral intake. After administration of intravenous glucose to further raise his blood sugar, the patient was advised by the physician to be more attentive in the management of his disease and was discharged home shortly thereafter.

Diabetes mellitus is a disease that results from the failure of an area of the pancreas called the Islets of Langerhans to produce a hormone called insulin. Insulin is responsible for allowing the passage of sugar from the bloodstream and into the cell where it can be utilized in the production of energy. Type I diabetes (insulin dependent) typically begins early in life, whereas type II diabetes (non-insulin dependent) is more prevalent in older people. In this particular case study, the patient was suffering from insulin shock as a result of hypoglycemia. The particular cause of this was explained within the flow of the case study. Hypoglycemia is a more common emergency complication in diabetic patients than is hyperglycemia (diabetic coma/diabetic ketoacidosis). The clinical presentation of the patient was consistent with one who had insufficient glucose to the brain. When this occurs, the signs and symptoms are extremely similar to that of a hypoxic patient, as the brain requires an adequate supply of sugar just as it does oxygen. Unmanaged hypoglycemia will ultimately result in permanent brain damage and cardiac arrest. It is important for the EMT to remember that a patient need not be a diabetic to become hypoglycemic. Prolonged heavy exercise and little to no oral intake can result in hypoglycemia as well.

EVALUATION

1. Which of the following signs is most consistent with hypoglycemia?
    a. warm, dry skin
    b. sudden onset
    c. slow onset
    d. excessive urination

2. Insulin is produced within which organ?
    a. pancreas
    b. liver
    c. spleen
    d. gallbladder

3. When receiving a call for a patient that is acting bizarrely, the EMT's priority is to:
    a. assume hypoglycemia and immediately administer glucose
    b. notify medical control to request permission to give sugar
    c. take measures that will ensure the safety of him and his crew
    d. treat the patient as though he is a psychiatric patient and notify the police

4. The patient with diabetic complications is most frequently mistaken for a patient that is:
    a. having a stroke
    b. intoxicated
    c. psychiatrically ill
    d. having a heart attack

5. A patient presents with an altered mental status. Her husband states that his wife took her insulin, but did not eat much. What is the most likely cause of her condition?

   a. diabetic coma
   b. diabetic shock
   c. insulin shock
   d. insulin coma

6. An insufficient supply of glucose to the brain will result in which of the following signs or symptoms?

   a. deep, rapid breathing
   b. tachycardia and a weak pulse
   c. bradycardia and hypertension
   d. excessive urination and thirst

7. A contraindication to the administration of oral glucose includes:

   a. a known history of diabetes
   b. a patient with an intact gag reflex
   c. the patient who is not alert enough to swallow
   d. uncertainty as to whether or not the blood sugar is high or low

8. Prior to administering oral glucose to a patient suspected of being hypoglycemic, the EMT should:

   a. begin transport of the patient
   b. perform a detailed physical exam
   c. make sure that the patient does not have a gag reflex
   d. verify the "five rights"

9. A patient with a history of type I diabetes presents with strange behavior and excessive hunger. He does not have an accu-check device and states that he has not checked his blood sugar in over a week. How should this patient be managed?

   a. transport only with continual monitoring
   b. assume hyperglycemia and withhold glucose
   c. contact medical control for authorization to administer glucose
   d. request an ALS unit to respond to the scene to administer insulin to the patient

10. An initial dose of oral glucose has been administered to a young female who is displaying classic signs and symptoms of hypoglycemia. As you reassess after the glucose, you note little change in her condition. You should:

    a. transport immediately
    b. request an ALS unit
    c. treat for hyperglycemia
    d. consider more oral glucose

15

I Am So Tired

Objectives

At the conclusion of this scenario, the participant will be able to:

1. Discuss causes of confusion in the geriatric patient.

2. Identify techniques for determining whether or not medications are being taken as prescribed.

3. Describe appropriate assessment and management techniques of a patient who is confused.

SCENARIO

Your ambulance has been dispatched to a residence on the outskirts of town. Dispatch reports that the caller, an elderly female, has stated that she is suddenly very tired and weak.

1. What are your thoughts concerning this dispatch information?

   Elderly patients may have many causes for feeling tired and weak. It may range from non-medical causes such as depression or loneliness to serious medical conditions such as cardiac or respiratory complications. Other causes may include anemia, low blood pressure, sepsis, and untoward effects of certain medications. You need to be prepared to do a thorough focused history and physical exam.

2. What should you do while en route to the call?

   You and your partner need to decide who will be responsible for the various functions of the call. You will also need to gather your body substance isolation (BSI) equipment, which should include gloves and eye protection.

You arrive on location. You grab your response bags and make way to the home. You remain very aware of scene safety during all aspects of the call. You knock on the door and you hear an elderly voice tell you to come in. You cautiously enter the home and are directed to the living area by the woman's voice. You see the woman sitting on a recliner. Her skin color looks pale. She asks if you are her son.

3. What information have you gained from this limited contact?

You have determined that the patient is conscious. You are concerned that she asked if you were her son. This could mean that the patient is confused. However, you must be aware that she is looking at you from across the room. Geriatric patients often have difficulty with vision. Do not assume that the patient is confused at this stage of the call.

You approach the patient and inform her that you are an EMT with the ambulance service and you are responding to her phone call for help. She says that she doesn't remember calling. You ask her if anything is wrong. She states that she is very tired and weak, which is not like her. Your initial assessment does not reveal any problems with the ABCs. She states that it all started yesterday and has gotten much worse today. You ask her if she has any pain and she denies having any. You ask if anyone lives with her and she tells you no. She does, however, have a son that comes by to check on her every evening. You ask if he came by last night but she can't recall. You begin your focused history and physical exam. The patient is conscious but disoriented as to date and place. She responds in confused statements. Her airway is open and patent. Her breathing is slightly fast but appears unlabored. She has a very weak and slow radial pulse, which you calculate to be 44. You direct your partner to begin oxygen administration at 4 Lpm with a nasal cannula.

4. What are your concerns based on this part of your survey?

Your major concern is that the patient has confusion. Confusion may have many causes such as dementia or Alzheimer's, but these are chronic diseases. Acute cases of confusion usually represent either inefficient delivery of blood or oxygen to the brain or cases involving ingestion of substances. Many medications, which are outside their therapeutic range, may also lead to alterations in mental status. Always assume that confusion is a new onset until proven otherwise. You should also be concerned about two items found on your assessment. You witnessed that the patient appeared pale in color. This is not uncommon in geriatric patients but it could represent poor perfusion of the skin. You have also found that the patient's heart rate is 44. A heart rate in the 40s is acceptable for a young athletic individual; however, it is probably not normal for a geriatric patient. This will require further investigation. The decreased heart rate and poor skin color are indications for calling advanced life support if available in your area.

You continue your assessment, which finds that the patient's pupils are equal, round, and reactive. She has no evidence of facial droop or slurring of the speech. Bilateral breath sounds are clear to auscultation. Her abdomen is slightly tender to palpation. She reports that she has gotten sick to her stomach twice today. You palpate no masses. Her extremities are unremarkable except for her skin color being pale and the slow heart rate. Assessment of her sensory and motor nervous system function is normal although she does have decreased strength. You direct your partner to perform vital signs as you attempt to gather a SAMPLE history.

You find that the patient can't remember if she is allergic to any medications. She does tell you that her medicines are on the kitchen table. She knows that she has had a heart problem for which she takes a medication. She is also on a medication for her blood pressure. She can't recall eating today and is very confused as to when all of this started.

5. What should you do now?

    Gather the medications that she is currently taking. Medications, if you refer to a drug guide, may help to inform you as to what medical condition the patient is being treated for. You should also assess the quantity of medication in the bottle and then look at the day it was prescribed and how often it is to be taken. On many occasions you will determine that the patient is either not taking the medication or taking it more or less often than prescribed. Many medications only work if the patient's blood level stays within a certain range. Therefore, medications that are not taken as prescribed may cause further problems. Another condition that may occur is termed polypharmacia. It occurs when patients have multiple medications from multiple physicians. They may not report a medication prescribed by one physician to the other physician because they believe that the medications are not related to their present complaint. Some drugs are dispensed under a trade name or under a generic name. If one physician prescribes Lasix and another prescribes Furosemide, the patient may not know he is taking two doses of the same drug. This can have lethal results.

You gather the medications, which are on the table. You see that one is a medication called Hydrochlorothiazide and the other is a medication called Digoxin. By looking at the bottle you see that the Digoxin is almost gone, but by the date of prescription she should have almost half of the bottle left. You ask the patient if she has been taking the small yellow pill as prescribed. She states that she is taking it twice a day like she thought she was supposed to. The bottle, however, is labeled for her to take the medication once per day. Your partner reports the following vital signs: B/P of 82/40, HR 44, RR 20, and an SpO_2 of 96 percent on oxygen. You assist the patient to the stretcher and secure her in position.

6. How do you determine if the medication she has taken too much of can cause a problem?

    You can refer to a drug reference handbook or you may wish to call poison control. Poison control is an excellent source of information regarding the effects of medications if taken in excess quantity. They will require some basic information such as the patient's age, weight, and signs or symptoms. You will also need to spell the medication for them and give them the date of prescription and the dose and quantity of medication taken.

    Digoxin (aka Lanoxin) is a cardiac glycoside. It is prescribed to improve the cardiac output of the heart. If given at correct doses it regulates the heart rate and provides for a more forceful contraction. However, Digoxin has a very narrow range of effectiveness. If levels are too low you do not see the beneficial effects. If the patient's level of Digoxin is too high it may become toxic. It causes a severe slowing of the heart and may also cause a decrease in blood pressure.

Hydochlorothiazide (aka HCTZ) is a thiazide diuretic. It is used in the treatment of hypertension. It works by increasing the removal of water from the vascular system by way of the kidneys. The reduction of water from the vascular system results in less blood pressure.

You decide to call poison control and give them their requested information. They inform you that she has indeed taken too much of the medication Digoxin. The side effects may include a slowing of the heart rate and a reduction of blood pressure. There is no antidote that you carry on your ambulance and medications such as activated charcoal are of no use since this was not a large, one-time ingestion. They recommend transport to the closest hospital for continued treatment.

You move the patient to the ambulance where you secure her for transport. Your partner begins driving to the hospital, which is approximately 10 minutes away. You continue the patient on oxygen and reassess her vital signs. You finish taking her blood pressure when suddenly she begins to dry heave as if to vomit.

7. What should your next action be?

Roll the patient onto her side. This is the quickest way to reduce the likelihood of her aspirating her own vomit. If the patient can't maintain her own airway you should use your Yankauer suction device and turn the suction unit on high. Remember to protect yourself from body substances. Try to avoid your exposure to the vomitus. You are probably very glad that you wore your eye protection on this call.

You suction the patient's oral cavity and remove any vomitus that is present. You were able to avoid exposure to your person during the event.

You continuously reassess your patient during the transport. You notify the hospital of your patient report via radio. The patient's condition remains unchanged during the transport. You deliver the patient to the emergency department where you give a full verbal report of your findings and interventions. You and your partner decontaminate the back of the ambulance after cleaning up the vomit. You complete your run form and return to service.

PATIENT OUTCOME/PATHOPHYSIOLOGY

The patient was evaluated in the emergency department. She was found to have a new onset of confusion secondary to a toxic level of Digoxin. She was initially treated with Kexalate enema in an attempt to remove some of the medication from her system. However, she continued to deteriorate so they were forced to place a breathing tube in the patient and begin mechanical ventilation. She then had large venous catheters placed in her femoral vein and underwent emergency dialysis to remove the toxic level of Digoxin. The dialysis was a success. She was subsequently taken off the breathing machine. She will be discharged in less than 7 days. It was the decision of her family that she be admitted to a long-term facility for geriatric clients to ensure that she gets the correct dosing of her medications.

1. Which of the following are causes of confusion in geriatric patients?
   a. dementia
   b. Alzheimer's
   c. medication toxicity
   d. hypotension
   e. all of the above

2. All geriatric patients should be assumed to be hard of hearing.
   a. true
   b. false

3. Which of the following is not likely to cause a patient to feel tired and weakened?
   a. loneliness
   b. depression
   c. cardiac complications
   d. hypertension

4. Which of the following is a complication caused by excessive levels of Digoxin?
   a. rapid heart rate
   b. hypertension
   c. slow heart rate
   d. tachypnea

5. What is the greatest risk of injury for geriatric patients?
   a. motor vehicle collision
   b. auto pedestrian collision
   c. falls
   d. assault

6. When patients have multiple medications from multiple physicians it may cause a condition known as:
   a. polyphagia
   b. polydipsia
   c. polypharmacia
   d. none of the above

7. If you suspect elder neglect or abuse you are legally required to report it.
   a. true
   b. false

8. People who are in the elderly age group have a large percentage of deaths caused by suicide.

   a. true
   b. false

9. Geriatric patients may be malnourished due to which of the following reasons?

   a. poor dental structures
   b. decreased appetite
   c. loneliness
   d. all of the above

10. Which of the following statements regarding geriatric patients is true?

   a. You should yell so that geriatric patients can hear you.
   b. Geriatric patients usually have a significant level of decreased mental function.
   c. Geriatric patients often lead active, vital lives.
   d. All of the above are true.

16

UNCONSCIOUS FEMALE

Objectives

At the conclusion of this scenario, the participant will be able to:

1. Recognize the signs and symptoms suggestive of a narcotic overdose.

2. Describe the assessment of the patient with a suspected narcotic overdose.

3. Define the principles of management for the patient with a narcotic overdose.

SCENARIO

It's Saturday night at approximately 2315 and you and your partner are watching the news when you are dispatched to the downtown area for a "man down." As you are responding, a police officer who is already on scene advises you that you have an "unconscious breathing female." You arrive at the scene, an apartment complex, where you see a crowd of people near one of the apartments. You cannot see the police officer.

1. What is your general impression of the scene?

   Because of the crowd and not knowing exactly what happened to the patient, your impression should be that of potential danger. What if the patient was shot and the "shooter" is one of those onlookers? Even though the police are on scene, you cannot see them. "Curious" onlookers can become a hostile crowd very quickly. You must take steps to remove these people from the scene, even if it means getting back on the radio, notifying the officer(s) on the scene, and having the people removed prior to your entry.

   Additional police officers arrive on the scene and disseminate the crowd of people. You approach the patient, a young female, who appears to be unconscious. At a glance, you see slight chest wall movement. One of the police officers recognizes the patient and tells you that she has been arrested in the past for drug possession. As you kneel down beside the patient, you glance at her arms.

2. What is your general impression of the patient?

    The unconsciousness and slight chest wall movement indicates a patient with inadequate breathing. Even though an initial assessment will still be performed, you know that this is a patient who will require ventilatory assistance.

3. What are you attempting to ascertain by looking at the patient's arms?

    Given the patient's present situation (unconscious with inadequate breathing) as well as her apparent criminal history of drug possession, you are looking specifically for needle tracks on her arms that would indicate habitual intravenous drug use.

Your initial assessment of the patient confirms her unresponsiveness. Her respirations are snoring, which you remedy with the proper airway maneuver. She is breathing shallowly at a rate of 6. Her heart rate is 52 and her skin is cool and moist. There is no apparent trauma or obvious bleeding that you can see.

4. What should you instruct your partner to do, based upon your findings in the initial assessment?

    Because you have not effectively ruled out trauma, you should direct your partner to stabilize the patient's head in a manual, in-line position and provide assisted ventilations with 100 percent oxygen. If the patient does not have a gag reflex, an oral airway should be inserted as well. Be sure to have suction available if needed.

5. How can the police be of assistance to you and your partner?

    The police can help you in several ways. First of all, because you are assuming this to be a potential trauma patient, you can direct an officer to retrieve your spinal precautions equipment from the ambulance. Another officer can question the bystanders in order to determine what might have happened to the patient. Bear in mind that you still need an officer to keep the onlookers at bay.

As your partner is providing the appropriate airway support for the patient, one of the police officers brings a young male to you, who states that the patient is his girlfriend and that she was "shooting up" in her apartment tonight. When she became unconscious, he moved her outside and laid her on the ground where she could get some fresh air. As the boyfriend is telling you this, you check the patient's pupils with your penlight.

6. How, if at all, will the information provided by the boyfriend affect your management of the patient?

    It will not affect your management of the patient in terms of airway management; however, it will serve to significantly increase your index of suspicion for a drug overdose. There are medications that can be administered by paramedics and at the hospital that can reverse the effects of certain drugs, but because this is beyond the scope of the EMT-B, prompt transport is important. The patient was removed from the apartment in a nontraumatic manner, so you can safely forego the spinal precautions.

7. Why look at the patient's pupils? What will this tell you?

There are several things that you can note by checking the patient's pupils. First of all, constricted or "pinpoint" pupils are indicative of a narcotic overdose and dilated or "blown" pupils indicate potential barbiturate overdose. This is important information for you to pass on to the receiving facility. Regardless of the type of drug the patient overdosed on, your management, specifically of the patient's airway, will still remain the same since both narcotics and barbiturates are central nervous system depressants and will suppress the patient's respirations.

You recognize the need for a rapid assessment of the patient due to the fact that she is unresponsive with inadequate breathing. During the assessment, you note the following:

- Airway still patent, respirations slow and shallow.
- Heart rate of 50 and weak at the radial pulse.
- Bruising along the veins of both of her arms (needle tracks).
- Pupillary constriction.
- A small bag with syringes and other paraphernalia strapped to her lower leg under her pants.

Continuing your management of the patient, you direct a police officer to the item on her leg, which he removes cautiously to prevent needlestick. Another officer has retrieved your ambulance stretcher for you.

8. Are there any legal issues that the EMT should be concerned with regarding this patient?

In general, drug overdoses in a known addict are not considered a "legally reportable case"; however, by pointing out the bag of apparent drug paraphernalia to the police officer, he will most likely want to question the boyfriend as to how and where it was obtained. Regardless of what is legally reportable or not, the EMT should always report suspicious findings to law enforcement or other appropriate personnel. It is important for the EMT to be aware of his legal obligations, as they vary from state to state.

The patient is loaded into the ambulance and transport to the hospital begins. You are busy in the back of the ambulance with your continued ventilatory assistance of the patient, so you ask your partner to radio ahead to the hospital with the patient information and estimated time of arrival.

9. As the single EMT in the back of the ambulance, what are your priorities of management with this patient?

Your priorities are that of continued airway management as well as preparation for the possibility of cardiopulmonary arrest. You can interrupt ventilations for up to 30 seconds to retrieve the AED and have it nearby in case this happens. Should the patient go into cardiac arrest, you would direct your partner to stop the ambulance and assist you in the back. Remember, the AED will not analyze in the back of a moving ambulance. Since you have been providing bag-valve mask ventilations on this patient for an extended period of time, a significant volume of air may accumulate in the stomach, increasing the risk of vomiting. If this happens, you will have to be prepared to turn the patient onto her side and provide suction.

After a transport time of approximately 12 minutes, you arrive at the emergency department and transfer care to the attending physician, while ventilatory assistance is continued. The physician immediately intubates the patient and orders lab work that will determine what the patient has overdosed on.

PATIENT OUTCOME/PATHOPHYSIOLOGY

After definitive airway management in the emergency department the patient was administered a medication called Narcan to reverse the effects of the heroin. Narcan is an opiate reversal agent that counteracts the effects of narcotic (opiate) drugs such as heroin, morphine, codeine, and demerol. After the administration of the Narcan, both her respirations and level of consciousness improved significantly. After 2 days in the hospital, she was transferred to a drug-addiction rehabilitation facility.

Heroin is a commonly abused drug. It is a powerful and highly addictive narcotic that is usually injected directly into a vein ("mainlined") to achieve its desired effect. Narcotics such as heroin are central nervous system depressants that suppress the patient's respirations, level of consciousness, blood pressure, and pulse. Significant amounts of heroin will depress the central nervous system to a point where cardiac arrest will result. In addition to the dangerous nature of the drug itself, it is typically self-administered with a "dirty" needle, which is the leading cause of the transmission of various communicable diseases, specifically HIV and hepatitis C.

EVALUATION

1. An overdose of a narcotic drug such as heroin will result in which of the following effects on the patient?

   a. hyperventilation

   b. hypertension

   c. bradycardia

   d. hyperactivity

2. A patient is suspected of having overdosed on a narcotic drug. He presents in a semiconscious state with respirations of 10 and shallow. Which of the following forms of airway management is appropriate for this patient?

   a. nonrebreather mask

   b. nasal airway and nonrebreather mask

   c. oral airway and nonrebreather mask

   d. oral airway and bag-valve mask device

3. A known drug addict is found unconscious and apneic on the floor of her living room. There were no witnesses to the event. Initial management includes all of the following EXCEPT:

   a. immediately assisting ventilations

   b. considering stabilization of the spine

c. performing a detailed physical exam

d. opening the airway with a head-tilt chin lift

4. After establishing an airway and assisting ventilations on a patient with a suspected narcotic overdose, the EMT should next:

   a. perform a rapid assessment

   b. look for needle tracks

   c. assess the patient's pulse

   d. transport without delay

5. Of the following medications, which is not a narcotic?

   a. heroin

   b. cocaine

   c. morphine

   d. demerol

6. You are summoned to a residence for a "drug overdose." When you arrive, a young female is frantically motioning for you to enter the house, stating that her boyfriend is unconscious. You note several people inside and one runs out the rear door. You respond appropriately by:

   a. immediately gaining access to the patient

   b. calling the police and then entering the house

   c. waiting for the police to secure the scene

   d. telling the woman to bring her boyfriend outside

7. Which of the following signs and symptoms are suggestive of narcotic overdose?

   a. bradycardia, hypertension, hypoventilation

   b. bradycardia, hypotension, hypoventilation

   c. tachycardia, dilated pupils, hyperventilation

   d. bradycardia, constricted pupils, hyperventilation

8. As an EMT-B, when managing a patient who has overdosed, you remember that legally, you must:

   a. report the overdose to the police department

   b. transport the patient to a drug rehabilitation center

   c. provide a consistently high standard of care

   d. administer Narcan if you carry it on the ambulance

9. You are transporting an overdose patient to a local hospital when the patient suddenly becomes pulseless and apneic. You should:

   a. attach the AED and initiate analysis of the patient's rhythm

   b. perform CPR and tell your partner to call the hospital

   c. have your partner stop the ambulance to assist you

   d. request an ALS ambulance and start CPR

10. Which of the following is the most reliable way to determine whether or not a patient has overdosed?

   a. looking for needle tracks

   b. checking the pupils for constriction

   c. performing a thorough history and exam

   d. asking any bystanders if the patient overdosed

17

MY DAUGHTER ATE MY MEDS

Objectives

At the conclusion of this scenario, the participant will be able to:

1. Identify risk factors for accidental pediatric toxic ingestions.

2. Discuss situations in which vomiting should or should not be induced.

3. Describe care of a pediatric patient suffering from a poisoning emergency.

SCENARIO

Your ambulance has been dispatched to a residence just outside the city limits. The caller, who is the patient's mother, reports that her 4-year-old has swallowed some of her medication. Dispatch states that the child is conscious and alert at the present time. Your ETA is 12 minutes.

1. What are your thoughts pertaining to this dispatch information?

    You are aware that your transport time will be slightly longer than usual because the call is taking place outside of the city. You are informed that you will be caring for a pediatric patient who is 4 years old. You realize that it will take a careful, professional approach to enlist the help of the patient and the parent. Unfortunately, you have not yet identified what type of medication was ingested. This would be helpful information if you could find out from the dispatcher. You would be able to contact poison control and get general information about the medication if the name were known. One positive piece of information that has been identified is that the child was awake and alert at the time of the call.

2. Can you identify risk factors that might lead to pediatric toxic ingestions?

There are several things that adults can do to decrease the risk of pediatric toxic ingestion. The most important thing that we could do is to safeguard our homes by childproofing them. You need to assess your home for poison exposure by taking a "child's eye view." This is much more beneficial than our adult view. Potential toxins need to be removed from the reach of children and the techniques they use to climb. Remove chemicals that will no longer be utilized. Child-proof cabinets and drawers. Prescribed medications should be stored in a secure cabinet that children do not have access to. Never attempt to administer medications to children by describing them as "candy." This makes children curious and may make them desire access to the medicine. We, as the public, should become active in legislating items such as candies that resemble medicines and vice versa. The best treatment for toxic ingestion is prevention.

During your response you and your partner decide which of you will perform what functions. You also gather your body substance isolation (BSI) equipment, which includes your gloves and eye protection.

You arrive on location. You and your partner are very aware of scene safety as you grab your response bags, pediatric kit, and your stretcher. You approach the home. You are met at the door and let in by the child's mother. She reports to you that her 4-year-old daughter climbed on top of the bathroom vanity and got her mother's bottle of medication. She took five tablets about 20–25 minutes ago. Mom called EMS because she didn't know what else to do.

She directs you to the child's room where she is sitting on the floor playing with some toys. The child is awake and alert to her mother and surroundings. You can see that her breathing appears unlabored and that she must have adequate circulation in order to sit and play as she is.

3. What should you do now?

You should gather more history from the mother. Information such as the patient's weight and any past medical problems would be helpful. You will need to ascertain the name of the medication she took, the number of pills/tablets, and the dose of said medication. Pinpoint the exact time of possible of ingestion. Remember to ask the mother if she did anything for the ingestion prior to your arrival. Many home remedies exist and you need to determine if any were employed.

You talk with mom regarding her daughter's SAMPLE history. You find that she is not allergic to any medications nor does she take any medications. She has no past medical problems and is up-to-date with all of her immunizations. You are informed that she last ate about 2 hours ago. Information about the ingestion is also gathered. The mother reports that her daughter took "no more than five of her antidepression pills." She is certain of the amount because she knew when she had to get her refill. The medication is called Elavil and each pill is 50 mg. You also find out that her daughter weighs about 40 lbs (18 Kg). The mother denies doing anything about the ingestion before your arrival. You also quickly assess the child with mom's presence and help. You find the child to be acting completely normal. She is awake, alert, and playful. Her LOC (Level/Loss of Consciousness), airway, breathing, and circulation are all normal. The physical exam finds that the patient's pupils are equal, round, and reactive. Breath sounds are clear to auscultation. Her abdomen is soft and she denies pain. Her extremities and back are unremarkable. Vital signs are B/P of 90/42, HR 96, and RR 20.

4. What should you do with this information?

You need to contact your poison control agency. You and your department should have your local number available to you at all times. Once contact has been made you will need to give the call-taker some important information. Poison control will ask you questions such as:

- Your name and whether you are a BLS or ALS provider
- Name of the patient
- Patient's age
- Patient's weight
- Medication taken
- Dosage of each pill/tablet
- Time of ingestion
- Was anything already given for the poison?
- Has the patient vomited?
- The findings of your physical assessment such as LOC and vital signs
- They will also want to know which hospital the patient will be taken to and how long your transport time will be

Ensure that you have all this information available so that it will expedite the call and give you the information you need.

5. Will you administer syrup of ipecac? Activated charcoal?

First, we will only administer these medications if instructed to do so by our medical director or standing order. Most physician medical directors will also require you to contact poison control to see if either of these medications is indicated.

Syrup of ipecac is an emetic. In other words it initiates vomiting. This was a mainstay of therapy for many years, until recently. Studies have shown that it may take as long as 20 or more minutes to initiate vomiting. Often more than one dose is required to achieve the result. The studies also concluded that patients only vomited between 25 and 30 percent of their stomach contents. Basically, it did not do an effective job in clearing the stomach. Also because of its time requirements, many of the poisons have already been absorbed by the body. If the patient had a change in level of consciousness before he vomited, then he would be subject to aspiration of stomach contents into the lungs. Because of these reasons, syrup of ipecac is seldom utilized. Many systems still keep it on the ambulance and in ERs for those rare occasions when it would be beneficial.

Activated charcoal is an adsorbent. This means that when it enters the stomach and gastrointestinal (GI) tract some poisons and medications will bind to it rather than being absorbed by the body. This allows many medications and other poisons to simply pass through the GI system without causing body damage. However, we would never give this medication if the patient ingested items such as acids, alkalis, toilet cleaners, drain cleaners, or lye. These poisons can literally eat holes in the esophagus, stomach, and intestines. Activated charcoal could then enter these erosions and damage the body further.

You contact poison control and give them a detailed report of your patient assessment and the information regarding the ingestion. They recommend that you do not give syrup of ipecac. Instead they suggest that the child receive 20 grams of activated charcoal by mouth and rapid transport to the hospital. They state that if the child becomes sleepy before or during the administration that you stop giving the medication. You are also instructed to be immediately ready to suction and clear the airway if she vomits and to have ventilation devices immediately available.

6. What information will you receive from poison control?

    Poison control will give you suggested guidelines about care. They are not authorized to give orders like medical control. If poison control suggests that you do a function, your medical control physician must still approve it.

    In this case they suggest 20 grams of activated charcoal. You carry both 20- and 25-gram doses. They tell you some information about the drug that was ingested:

    Elavil (aka Amitriptyline) is a medication known as a tricyclic antidepressant. With overdoses you would expect to see a gradual and then sudden decrease in level of consciousness, which could lead to coma or death. Vital signs will be altered with an increase in heart rate and a decrease in blood pressure. It may also interrupt the normal cardiac activity of the heart, which could lead to cardiac arrest.

You ask mom to get the child's favorite cup, preferably one with a lid and a straw. After the mother returns with the cup you ask her to carry the child to the ambulance so that she will not be so frightened. You explain what poison control said about the medication and that you need to get to the hospital in a quick and safe manner.

While en route you contact your medical control physician and she orders you to administer the 20 grams of activated charcoal by mouth and to begin blow-by oxygen if the child will tolerate it.

7. How will you prepare and then administer the activated charcoal?

    Activated charcoal is a very thick and black substance that does not appear appetizing to adults, much less children. You will need to disguise the administration process by hiding it. It should be placed in a cup with a lid and simply encourage, or have mom or dad encourage, the child to sip the medication. Because activated charcoal is so thick you will need to shake it extremely well before pouring it into the cup.

8. What will you need to prepare in the back of the ambulance?

    Remember what poison control instructed. You will need to turn on your suction and have it immediately available. You will also want to prepare a pediatric bag-valve mask device and also have available an appropriately sized oropharyngeal airway. This child's breathing may be interrupted without warning. Be prepared to breathe for the child.

You ask the patient's mother to direct the blow-by oxygen, which the child seems to tolerate. She is also sipping the activated charcoal very slowly but is responding to Mom's encouragement to continue.

You give a radio report to the receiving hospital while en route. The child continues to remain unchanged during the transport to the hospital. You are able to reassess and perform repeat vital signs as well. She remains stable throughout. Upon arrival at the Children's Hospital you transfer the patient and her mother to the emergency department. You give the staff a complete report of your findings and note that the child did completely take the 20 grams of activated charcoal. You and your partner depart the ER and prepare your ambulance for the next call.

PATIENT OUTCOME/PATHOPHYSIOLOGY

The child was admitted to the ER of Children's Hospital. She was diagnosed with an accidental ingestion of 250 mg of Elavil. She was admitted to the pediatric ICU, where she began to suffer a decreased level of consciousness and vital sign changes. She had a breathing tube placed and mechanical ventilation was initiated. She received IV fluids in conjunction with numerous medications. She began to improve after several days of treatment. She was eventually taken off the breathing machine. Her vital signs have all returned to normal. Liver and kidney functions have also returned to normal. She will be discharged to home in several days.

EVALUATION

1. An emetic is something that will induce:
   a. constipation
   b. diarrhea
   c. vomiting
   d. food absorption

2. Which of the following initiates a patient to vomit?
   a. syrup of ipecac
   b. Elavil
   c. activated charcoal
   d. none of the above

3. Which of the following causes certain poisons and medications to bind to its components?
   a. syrup of ipecac
   b. Elavil
   c. activated charcoal
   d. none of the above

4. Which of the following preventive techniques should have the highest priority?
   a. labeling bottles
   b. moving all medications to higher shelves
   c. hiding cleaning agents
   d. "childproofing" the home

5. You should not administer activated charcoal to patients who have ingested which of the following poisons?

    a. drain cleaner

    b. toilet cleaners

    c. lye

    d. all of the above

6. Which of the following reasons have led to the reduced use of syrup of ipecac?

    a. cost of the medication

    b. may be harmful to utilize syrup-based medications in diabetics

    c. it only clears the stomach of 30 percent of its contents

    d. short shelf life

7. When syrup of ipecac is administered, you would expect to see vomiting in:

    a. 10 minutes

    b. 20 minutes

    c. 30 minutes

    d. 40 minutes

8. Which of the following is information required by poison control?

    a. patient's weight

    b. time of ingestion

    c. how much medication taken

    d. where the patient will be transported to

    e. all of the above

9. If medication is suggested by poison control you should give it without contacting medical control.

    a. true

    b. false

10. It is imperative to administer activated charcoal to patients even though they have a decreased level of consciousness.

    a. true

    b. false

18

I Think We Have the Flu

Objectives

At the conclusion of this scenario, the participant will be able to:

1. Describe the assessment techniques for a responsive medical patient.

2. Define the signs and symptoms of carbon monoxide poisoning.

3. Describe the management of the patient with carbon monoxide poisoning.

SCENARIO

Your unit is dispatched to a residence approximately 5 miles from your station for a 53-year-old female and her 56-year-old husband, both of whom are complaining of a headache, nausea, and vomiting. It is approximately 30° outside, as the season's first cold front has just passed. The time of call is 0310.

You arrive at the scene and enter the house. You find the wife sitting at the kitchen table. There is a bowl in her lap that she has been vomiting in. Her husband walks into the kitchen complaining of the same symptoms and states, "I think we have the flu."

1. How will you manage these patients initially?

Because both of the patients are responsive, you and your partner should each pick a patient and complete your initial assessments, which would include assessing the airway and breathing. Also assess the rate, regularity, and quality of pulse as well as assessing skin color, condition, and temperature. You will also determine the patients' chief complaints.

The wife advises you that she got up to go to the bathroom when she noticed the symptoms. Her husband heard her vomiting and woke up; he then realized that he wasn't feeling well either.

2. What is the correlation, if any, between the weather and the patient's symptoms?

   When people turn on their gas heaters for the first time of the season, temperature changes throughout the year that caused small cracks in the heater line allow gas to escape.

3. What relationship might this have to the patient's symptoms?

   Exposure to carbon monoxide gas could certainly explain the symptoms that the patients are experiencing. It is too coincidental that they should both happen to develop the flu at the same time. Typically, the flu affects one of the family members, who passes it along to another, whose symptoms usually appear 12 to 24 hours later.

4. What is your priority of management for these two patients?

   Get them, as well as you and your partner, out of the house immediately! Place them in the ambulance and complete the remainder of your assessment and initiate any management. It is clear that gasses from the heater are to blame for the patient's symptoms.

Once in the ambulance, you initiate 100 percent oxygen via nonrebreather mask for both patients and continuously monitor their airways in case they vomit again. Their vital signs are within normal limits for their age groups. In obtaining the SAMPLE history on both patients, the only remarkable finding is that the husband has a history of angina pectoris, which is managed with nitroglycerin. He states that he hasn't had an episode of chest pain in over 3 months.

5. Are there any other considerations in addition to removing the patients from the house?

   Notification of the fire department should be made to safely ventilate the house and shut down the heater. The fire department and/or power company will also have a meter available to measure gas levels in the residence.

6. Of what benefit will 100 percent oxygen be to these patients?

   Considering that the gas that was leaking from this family's heater contained carbon monoxide (accounting for their symptoms), oxygen is more beneficial that any other field treatment that can be rendered. Carbon monoxide causes a separation of hemoglobin and oxygen, which inhibits the overall processes of oxygenation and perfusion. A constant supply of supplemental oxygen must be administered to these patients until more definitive care can be given.

You hand the husband an emesis basin as he begins to vomit. You request that they allow you to transport them to the hospital. They agree and state that they wish to go to their "family hospital," which is a 12 to 15 minute drive away. City public service and the fire department are now on the scene and have secured the environment. You begin transport to the hospital of the patient's choice.

7. What additional treatment will these patients possibly require that cannot be provided by EMS or the emergency department?

Definitive care for patients suffering from carbon monoxide poisoning is a hyperbaric chamber, which will depend upon the concentration of carbon monoxide in their blood. The patients will receive arterial blood gas analysis in the emergency department to make that determination.

With an estimated time of arrival to the emergency department of 5 minutes, you call in your patient report. You advise the nurse taking your report of the patients' complaints as well as the environment in which they were found. While briefly glancing at both patients' skin color, you report their vital signs and the fact that they are both on 100 percent oxygen via nonrebreather masks. The nurse acknowledges your report.

8. Why glance at their skin color? What are you looking for?

Because carbon monoxide molecules are bright red in color, you are evaluating the patients for the classic "cherry red" skin color seen in severe cases of carbon monoxide poisoning. It must be pointed out that although this is a classic sign, it is also a very rare and late sign. Patients with carbon monoxide poisoning will develop cyanosis due to the inhibition of oxygenation long before their skin turns red. The vast majority of patients who develop cherry red skin will be in critical condition (many do not exhibit it until after death).

Both patients are received at the emergency department in unchanged condition. After a brief update with the nurse who took your radio report, you and your partner return to service.

PATIENT OUTCOME/PATHOPHYSIOLOGY

Upon arterial blood gas analysis, both patients were found to have had significant amounts of carbon monoxide in their blood. They were transferred to a local Air Force hospital having a hyperbaric chamber. After 4 hours in the chamber, their symptoms resolved. Further analysis of their blood revealed no carbon monoxide residue. They were monitored for a short time in the emergency department and discharged. They were also advised not to return to their house until the gas heater could be repaired. They wholeheartedly agreed.

Carbon monoxide (CO), which is produced by the incomplete combustion of many chemicals and products such as wood and fabric, is a colorless, odorless, and tasteless gas. It has an affinity for hemoglobin 250 times greater than that of oxygen. This means that it will force the oxygen away from the hemoglobin molecule and prevent oxygenation. People who die of CO poisoning usually do so in their sleep unless awakened by symptoms. The level of carbon monoxide in our blood should be "0"; however, due to the smokers around us, as well as the exhaust from automobiles (most common), we all have small, nontoxic amounts of it in our blood (normally < 0.1 percent). Carbon monoxide poisonings, with the exception of those who commit suicide by sitting in their running automobiles in the garage, tend to be seasonal in occurrence, typically during the early part of winter as people run their gas heaters for the first time of the season. Initial management for CO-poisoned patients includes 100 percent oxygen. Definitive management includes placing the patient in a hyperbaric chamber, which, through the use of pressurized oxygen, forces the carbon monoxide away from the hemoglobin, thereby allowing the reuniting of oxygen.

EVALUATION

1. What effect does carbon monoxide have on the blood?
   a. it binds with the white blood cell
   b. it binds with the red blood cell
   c. it binds with oxygen molecules
   d. it binds with hemoglobin molecules

2. Typical signs and symptoms of carbon monoxide poisoning include which of the following?
   a. cherry red skin color
   b. severe headache
   c. severe muscle spasm
   d. loss of vision in one eye

3. Initial management for a patient suspected of being exposed to carbon monoxide includes:
   a. 100 percent oxygen via nonrebreather mask
   b. rapid transport to a hyperbaric chamber
   c. removing the patient from the environment
   d. placing the patient in the shock position

4. Which of the following best describes the characteristics of carbon monoxide?
   a. it emits a greenish fog
   b. it emits a purplish fog
   c. it smells like rotten eggs
   d. it cannot be tasted

5. Carbon monoxide has an affinity for the molecule that it targets that is _____ times greater than that of oxygen.
   a. 100
   b. 150
   c. 250
   d. 500

6. A classic but late sign of carbon monoxide poisoning is:
   a. nausea and vomiting
   b. cyanosis to the face
   c. cherry red skin color
   d. an occipital headache

7. Which of the following patients should be suspected of suffering from carbon monoxide poisoning?

    a. a sudden onset of chest pain while watching TV

    b. awakens in the middle of a summer night with a headache

    c. complains of severe nausea during the early part of winter

    d. severe leg cramps after taking a prolonged nap in the fall

8. Which of the following would be more suggestive of carbon monoxide poisoning versus the flu?

    a. vomiting and fever in multiple family members

    b. severe headache in multiple family members

    c. two patients complain of chest pain 24 hours apart

    d. all of these are suggestive of carbon monoxide poisoning

9. What is the most common producer of carbon monoxide on a daily basis?

    a. cigarette smoke

    b. leaks in a heater line

    c. automobile exhaust

    d. structural fires

10. What should be the EMT's immediate concern when applying oxygen by non-rebreather mask to a patient with suspected carbon monoxide poisoning?

    a. the patient will not tolerate the mask

    b. the patient may vomit and aspirate

    c. the oxygen may make the headache worse

    d. the patient may develop an altered mental state

19

DIZZY AND WEAK

Objectives

At the conclusion of this scenario, the participant will be able to:

1. Define the various types of heat-related emergencies.

2. Describe the assessment of the patient with a heat-related emergency.

3. Describe the management of the patient with a heat-related emergency.

SCENARIO

On a hot and humid summer day, you receive a call to a local park for a male patient complaining of nausea, lightheadedness, and generalized weakness. The time of the call is 1430. You arrive on the scene at 1440, where the patient is found sitting on a park bench talking to a bystander. His appearance is pale and he is sweating profusely. He is near an adjacent area of trees.

1. What is your general impression of this patient?

    Your impression of the patient is that of one who is conscious and oriented. He speaks without evidence of respiratory distress. With this, you have essentially completed a significant portion of your initial assessment. The pallor and diaphoresis could indicate a variety of problems including, but not limited to:

    - AMI
    - Anaphylaxis
    - Diabetic problems
    - Environmental emergency

2. Are there any special considerations or actions that you should take with regard to the patient's general appearance and location?

Clearly because of the heat and the fact that the patient is sitting right in the middle of it, he should be immediately moved to a cooler area, whether it is under the adjacent trees or in the back of your ambulance. If moved to the ambulance, be sure to turn on the air conditioner. Any of the potential problems mentioned earlier could be made worse by the heat.

You relocate the patient, who is 24 years old, to the ambulance and begin your initial assessment. The patient's airway is clear. He is speaking full sentences without respiratory distress. His pulse is weak at the radial site at a rapid rate and his respirations are slightly shallow at 28. His skin is cool and moist to the touch. He states that he feels nauseated, is "weak all over," and is very thirsty. He further tells you that he has been flying his remote control airplane for the past 3 hours.

3. What have you learned from the initial assessment as well as the patient's chief complaint?

This patient has been in a hot environment for an extended period of time. Though his signs and symptoms suggest a heat emergency with dehydration, you must still gather additional information in an attempt to establish the cause of these signs and symptoms. As previously mentioned, a variety of illnesses can manifest with this type of presentation.

4. What will your management consist of? Any special considerations?

Because you have already moved the patient to a cooler environment, it would be appropriate to apply oxygen and further cool the patient (removing clothing and fanning the patient). You must also be prepared to treat the patient for shock due to the significant fluid loss. If he becomes unconscious, as patients with his problem may do, airway management will be a high priority. As you are managing the patient, a focused history and physical exam can be obtained.

There is one statement that the patient made that will affect your management. He stated that he is nauseated. With this in mind, you might want to apply oxygen with a nasal cannula in case he vomits. Additionally, patients who are nauseated and thirsty should not be given anything to drink as this would most likely result in vomiting and the risk of aspiration.

As your partner obtains a set of baseline vital signs, you render the appropriate management and begin a focused history and physical exam of the patient. The findings are as follows:

- O—the onset of symptoms was gradual.
- P—the longer he stayed in the heat, the worse he felt.
- Q—his nausea is becoming progressively severe.
- R—he has no pain (not applicable).
- S—he states that he feels "very bad."
- T—the symptoms began approximately 45 minutes ago.

His baseline vital signs are B/P 100/60 and pulse 130 (lying down). His respirations are 26 and slightly shallow.

5. With his history and vital signs reinforcing your suspicion of dehydration, is there any way that you could determine the severity?

A patient with a "resting tachycardia" and a history of prolonged exposure to the heat suggests significant dehydration in and of itself. Orthostatic vital signs can be obtained to determine the severity of his dehydration. To do this, you take the patient's blood pressure and pulse in a seated/lying position, and then you stand the patient up for approximately 2 minutes and repeat the vital signs. A decrease in the patient's systolic blood pressure by 15 mmHg or more and/or a heart rate increase by 15 beats per minute or more is considered "orthostasis" and suggests significant dehydration. The EMT must be very careful if he elects to perform this test, especially in patients who are lightheaded or dizzy. If the patient stands up too fast, he could faint; if the EMTs are not there to support him, injury to the patient could result. Orthostatic vital signs are usually obtained when determining whether or not intravenous rehydration is indicated (not an EMT-B skill). Refer to your locally established protocols with regard to obtaining orthostatic vital signs.

You discuss your findings with the patient and advise him that he needs to be transported to the hospital for further evaluation. He tells you that he will probably be okay and that he really does not wish to go to the hospital. He says that he will go home and rest for a couple of hours.

6. What suggestions would you make to this patient based upon his desire not to be transported to the hospital?

You should explain the situation and potential complications to the patient and again request that he allow you to transport him. Due to the fact that the patient is significantly dehydrated, he needs intravenous fluid rehydration, which is beyond your scope of practice and can only be provided in the hospital. In addition, because of his lightheadedness, you should be concerned with his ability to drive. Although the patient is legally able to refuse transport (he is conscious and alert and over 18 years of age), he must be made aware of the potential ramifications of transport refusal. If he maintains his decision not to be transported, he should be advised as follows:

- Do not drive. Call someone to drive him home.
- Have someone stay with him for a while.
- Remain in a cool environment for the rest of the day.
- Call 911 if he begins to feel worse.

Remember, it is your legal responsibility to ensure that patients refusing treatment and/or transport are aware of the possible consequences of their refusal. Thorough documentation of this is important. A signed refusal must be obtained for patients refusing EMS treatment/transport.

After a few minutes of convincing, the patient agrees to ambulance transport to the hospital. Your partner prepares the stretcher as you comment on the wise decision that the patient has made.

En route to the hospital, the patient's condition remains essentially unchanged. You repeat his vital signs and continually monitor him. He is delivered to the emergency department staff and a report is given to the nurse in charge.

PATIENT OUTCOME/PATHOPHYSIOLOGY

The patient was diagnosed in the emergency department with heat exhaustion and significant dehydration. He was given intravenous fluids, monitored for 3 hours, and discharged home with instructions to remain out of the heat for the next few days.

Heat exhaustion is a reaction that results from a prolonged exposure to a hot environment. It is the most common heat-related illness seen by the EMT. With prolonged exposure to heat, patients will begin to lose water and sodium (salt) from the body as their core body temperature rises. Recall that one of the ways the body will attempt to maintain a normal core temperature is through sweating, which results in a loss of sodium and eventual dehydration, which explains the signs and symptoms of heat exhaustion (weak and rapid pulse, thirst, lightheadedness, etc.). Failure to effectively manage heat exhaustion will result in the patient developing heatstroke, a dire emergency in which the body is seriously depleted of sodium and water. With no way for the body to remove heat through sweating, the core body temperature will soar, which could result in permanent brain damage or death.

EVALUATION

1. Immediate care for a patient with a heat-related illness includes:
   a. applying 100 percent oxygen
   b. moving the patient to a cool area
   c. rapid cooling by any means possible
   d. giving the patient cold fluids to drink

2. Signs of heat exhaustion include which of the following?
   a. hot, dry skin
   b. warm, moist skin
   c. cool, moist skin
   d. cool, dry skin

3. A 22-year-old patient presents with dizziness, nausea, and a heart rate of 140 after 4 hours of heavy exercise in 95° heat. You should:
   a. give the patient fluids to drink
   b. start an IV to rehydrate the patient
   c. remove the patient from the hot environment
   d. place the patient in a prone position and give oxygen

4. Orthostatic vital signs are obtained in order to:
   a. determine the severity of dehydration
   b. determine whether the patient is injured
   c. differentiate between heat cramps and heatstroke
   d. determine whether or not transport is necessary

5. A patient is considered orthostatic if his heart rate:
   a. decreases by 15 beats/min. or more upon standing
   b. increases by 15 beats/min. or more upon standing
   c. decreases by 15 beats/min. or more upon lying
   d. increases by 15 beats/min. or more upon lying

6. Which of the following treatment regimens would be least appropriate for a patient with suspected heat exhaustion who is complaining of nausea?
   a. obtaining orthostatic vital signs
   b. applying oxygen via nasal cannula
   c. transporting to the hospital for rehydration
   d. giving the patient cold fluids by mouth

7. You are managing a young female with a heat-related illness when she suddenly loses consciousness. The EMT should first:
   a. initiate rapid cooling immediately
   b. ensure that her airway is patent
   c. apply oxygen with a nonrebreather mask
   d. suction the patient's oropharynx

8. A patient with heat exhaustion refuses ambulance transport to the hospital. What advice should the EMT give to her?
   a. wait 1 to 2 hours before returning to prior activities
   b. drive herself to the hospital if needed
   c. stay out of the heat for at least 24 hours
   d. drink plenty of fluids if she becomes nauseated

9. The primary mechanism that the body uses in order to release heat from the body is to:
   a. breathe faster
   b. sweat/perspire
   c. increase urine output
   d. increase the heart rate

10. Signs of dehydration include all of the following EXCEPT:
    a. lightheadedness
    b. resting tachycardia
    c. increased blood pressure
    d. excessive thirst

20

FEELING WEAK AT A NURSING HOME

Objectives

At the conclusion of this scenario, the participant will be able to:

1. Discuss common causes of weakness and dizziness in geriatric patients.

2. Identify signs and symptoms of gastrointestinal (GI) bleeding.

3. List ways of determining the difference between lower- and upper-GI bleeding.

SCENARIO

Your ambulance has been dispatched to a nursing home for a patient complaining of being weak and dizzy. Your ETA is 5 minutes.

1. What are your thoughts concerning this dispatch information?

    Geriatric patients may have numerous causes for the complaint of being weak and dizzy. They range from heart conditions such as abnormal beats to congestive heart failure. Other causes include breathing problems that interfere with oxygenation and exhalation of waste products. Electrolyte imbalances may also lead to this feeling. Anemia, or low blood count, may be a consideration as well.

2. What should you do while en route to this call?

    You and your partner need to decide who will perform the different tasks and functions during this call. You will also need to gather your personal protective equipment, which should include gloves and eye protection at a minimum.

    You arrive on location, where you are directed to the far end of a hallway. Mrs. Johnson is an 88-year-old patient who has resided in the nursing home for about 3 years. You make your way to her room where you find nursing assistants giving her a bath and changing her gown. You note that the patient appears pale in color. You approach and begin your focused history and physical exam. You note that the patient is conscious but somewhat confused about her location and the date. One of the staff members tells you that she is normally pretty alert but has deteriorated today. You determine that her airway is open and patent. She is breathing 28/minute with some occasional coughing noted. Her radial pulse is weak and very rapid at approximately 140/minute. You also note that her capillary refill is delayed and is about 4 seconds.

3. What are your thoughts regarding the information gained during your primary survey?

This patient is critically ill. She displays numerous signs of shock. She is disoriented, has a rapid heart rate, rapid breathing, delayed capillary refill, and poor skin color. This is a true emergency. The things you have noted are not normal for anyone, including someone who resides in a nursing home.

4. What are your first interventions?

Direct your partner to begin oxygen administration and place the patient in a shock position. You will begin your assessment to see if you can determine the cause of shock as you prepare for immediate transport. You will also need someone from the facility to give you pertinent medical information and records, which should include information regarding resuscitation status.

You direct your partner to begin oxygen administration at 15 Lpm with a nonrebreather mask. You also place pillows under the patient's lower legs to aid in shock management. You request that someone who has information about the patient come to the room. One of the aides tells you that they will go get the registered nurse (RN). You begin your physical exam while waiting for the staff. The patient's LOC remains unchanged. She is alert but not aware of her location or the date. Her ABCs also remain unchanged. You find that her lips appear pale. Pupils are unequal but you note a cataract in the left eye. You note that she has a medication patch on her right anterior chest, which is labeled "nitroglycerin." Auscultation of breath sounds reveals that she has diffuse coarse rhonchi, which are improved by her coughing. Her abdomen is soft and no palpable masses are noted. Her lower extremities are cool to the touch and are slightly mottled distally. You also note a well-healed surgical scar to her left hip region. No pedal pulses are noted but the patient does move both feet spontaneously. Upper extremities are also pale and cool to the touch. Weak radial pulses are noted and the patient will grip your hands upon request. As you turn the patient to examine her back you see that she has been incontinent of stool. You note that it is dark black in color, almost tar-like. It also has a foul odor. You direct your partner to assess vital signs.

5. What is the significance of her stool color?

Black, tar-like stools are usually indicative of a gastrointestinal (GI) bleed. Blood that passes through the GI tract undergoes the same attempts at digestion as does food. Chemicals and bacteria try to break down the blood and cause it to change colors and develop a foul smell.

6. What causes this?

This GI bleed is occurring somewhere high in the intestines. The closer the bleeding site is to the rectum the less time it is exposed to digestive processes. This would mean that lower-GI bleeding usually displays visible blood. The higher the bleeding site the more black and tar-like the stool will be. In this case we have a high-GI bleed. This may be caused by conditions such as diverticulitis, tumors, ulcers, and chronic diseases such as irritable bowel and Chron's disease.

The nurse arrives in the room as you and your partner are moving the patient to the stretcher. The nurse apologizes for getting here so late because she has another very sick person in another hall. She is the only RN in the building and cares for sixty patients. She informs you that Mrs. Johnson has developed a black, tar-like stool since yesterday. They did a guiac test for occult blood and it was positive. She has progressively gotten worse today and is to be a direct admit to the hospital. Her medical records reveal that she is allergic to penicillin. She presently has a list of medications, which includes Digoxin, nitroglycerin patch, multivitamins, and Tylenol. Her past medical history includes two previous myocardial infarctions and a fracture and repair of the left hip. Your partner reports the following vital signs: B/P of 78/38, HR 140, RR of 28, SpO_2 of 95 percent on oxygen and capillary refill of 4 seconds. The nurse verbalizes that she is getting worse and very rapidly.

7. What should you do for these vital signs?

This patient was suspected to be in shock based upon your assessment. The vital signs reinforce your suspicion. You will continue to administer oxygen and assist respirations if necessary. You will also keep the patient in a shock-management position with the lower extremities elevated. You will cover her with a blanket in an attempt to keep her body temperature normal. You should also be familiar with the effects of the medication she is receiving.

The RN states that with a blood pressure that low she should remove her nitroglycerin patch to aid in blood pressure maintenance.

You and your partner quickly transport the patient to the ambulance and begin emergency transport to the hospital. Your ETA is 4 minutes. You continue to provide oxygen administration and reassess vital signs en route. You deliver the patient to the hospital where she is admitted to the floor area. Upon seeing the patient, the doctor tells you not to take her off the stretcher and to follow him to the ICU. During the walk to the unit you are able to give a complete report to the physician. You deliver the patient to the unit where you repeat your report to the nursing staff. You then return to your ambulance and prepare for the next call.

MEDS

Digoxin (aka Lanoxin) is a cardiac glycoside. This means that it improves the effectiveness of each cardiac contraction and regulates its rate. This will keep the heart in a steady rhythm and increase its pumping function.

Tylenol (aka acetaminophen) is an analgesic and antipyretic. Simply put, it reduces pain and fever.

Multivitamins are a compilation of vitamins and minerals to supplement daily oral intake of food products, which may be insufficient.

Nitroglycerin (aka Nitrodur) may be administered by tablets, continuous IV infusion, or by the transdermal method (as in the case of this patch). Nitroglycerin causes vasodilatation, which helps to reduce blood pressure and keep coronary arteries open.

After looking at these medications you can see any further intervention that may be employed. You may need to have permission from the physician to do this. You should remove the nitroglycerin patch or ask the RN to remove the medication. This patient is already in shock with a low blood pressure. The continuous administration of nitroglycerin will not help the situation.

PATIENT OUTCOME/PATHOPHYSIOLOGY

The patient was admitted to the ICU with the diagnosis of an upper-GI bleed. She received multiple units of blood but despite aggressive therapy she did not recover from this event. She died the following day.

EVALUATION

1. Stools from upper-GI bleeds are commonly described as:
   a. chalk-like in color
   b. blood colored
   c. black, tar-like
   d. brown colored

2. Stools from lower-GI bleeds are commonly described as:
   a. chalk-like in color
   b. blood colored
   c. black, tar-like
   d. brown colored

3. Which of the following are causes of GI bleeds?
   a. ulcers
   b. inflammatory bowel
   c. tumors
   d. all of the above

4. A capillary refill of less than _____ seconds is normal in an adult patient.
   a. 1
   b. 2
   c. 3
   d. 4

5. Rhonchi are often described as:
   a. coarse, wet breath sounds
   b. fine, moist breath sounds
   c. musical breath sounds
   d. crowing breath sounds

6. Nitroglycerin may lower the patient's blood pressure.
   a. true
   b. false

7. Unequal pupils may be caused by which of the following?
   a. closed head injury
   b. cataract
   c. common in 10 percent of the population
   d. all of the above

8. Confusion in geriatric patients may be caused by which of the following?
   a. dementia
   b. Alzheimer's
   c. shock
   d. all of the above

9. You as an EMT are allowed to take orders from a registered nurse.
   a. true
   b. false

10. All patients admitted to a nursing home have "do not resuscitate" orders upon admission.
    a. true
    b. false

21

I Am Having Problems Swallowing

Objectives

At the conclusion of this scenario, the participant will be able to:

1. Describe signs and symptoms of an allergic reaction.

2. Discuss complications that can occur secondary to anaphylaxis.

3. List treatment options for partial airway obstructions secondary to soft tissue swelling.

SCENARIO

Your ambulance has been dispatched to a residence for an adult female who called because she is having problems swallowing. She informed the dispatcher that she is concerned that she may be having a reaction to medication.

1. What are your thoughts concerning this dispatch information?

   You were informed that you have an adult female who is having difficulty swallowing. There are several causes for difficulty with swallowing, such as food bolus obstruction of the esophagus, difficulty swallowing from a stroke, and soft tissue swelling often associated with an allergic reaction. This caller also states that she believes she is reacting to a medication. If so, then this caller may experience a serious allergic reaction.

2. What is the most significant complication of medication allergies?

   Death. Death from a medication allergy is possible if the patient suffers the most severe form of an allergic reaction. This type of a reaction is termed "anaphylaxis." Anaphylaxis is a condition that leads to circulatory and respiratory collapse. In some cases anaphylaxis causes a swelling of the airways that will completely obstruct the airway. This may happen alone or in conjunction with shock secondary to loss of vascular tone and leakage of fluid from the capillary system. Anaphylaxis requires prompt treatment to prevent severe complications. It is caused by an immune response to a foreign matter that enters the circulatory system. This may be caused by items such as venoms from insects, inhaled chemicals such as perfumes or scents, foods such as those containing peanuts, and medications such as antibiotics. There are numerous items that can cause an allergic reaction. We term the item that causes the immune response an "allergen." Anaphylaxis is actually an attempt to clear an allergen, which can cause the person's own death.

You arrive on scene. You gather your equipment as you put on your body substance isolation (BSI) equipment. You are very observant as you approach the home to ensure your safety. You knock on the door but no one answers. You look through the screen and you are able to see an adult female sitting on the floor of the kitchen area. She is reaching out. You call to see if she can answer or come to the door but she is unable to talk back to you.

3. What should you do next?

    You should radio dispatch that you are making an entry and that they should send law enforcement. You must assume that the woman's inability to communicate represents a serious medical problem. As always, remain very aware of the scene and the potential for danger.

You enter the residence and approach the woman sitting on the floor. You are able to see that she is cyanotic and appears very apprehensive.

4. What have you learned from this brief encounter?

    This is a true emergency. This patient is in a severe form of respiratory distress. Cyanosis is a late sign of respiratory compromise. In order for the patient to be cyanotic, greater than 50 percent of her hemoglobin must lack oxygen binding to it. You will need to identify the cause and make an attempt at early intervention.

You immediately direct your partner to administer oxygen at 15 Lpm with a nonrebreather mask as you begin your patient assessment. You ask the patient what is the matter and if she is hurting. You see that she is having great difficulty breathing and can't even speak because of it. She points to a medication that is setting on the counter. Your partner picks up the bottle and reads the name: Amoxicillin. You continue to assess the patient. You have already identified that she is conscious. Her airway is open but she is making stridorous sounds as she breaths. Her tongue and lips appear swollen. She is breathing very shallow and rapidly and is using most all of her accessory muscles. You check her pulse and find that she has a very rapid and weak radial pulse.

5. What should your next intervention be?

    You should begin to package the patient for load-and-go transport. You have identified that this is a serious condition and one that cannot be managed in the field. Anaphylaxis requires emergent medication administration. You should begin immediate transport to the closest hospital and call for an ALS ambulance or supervisor to meet you en route.

NOTE: *An increasing number of BLS ambulances are carrying epinephrine autoinjectors. If you have an autoinjector available it would be appropriate to contact medical control to obtain permission for its use. Prompt transport and ALS intercept are also still appropriate, even with the use of the epinephrine.*

You and your partner immediately place the patient on the stretcher and seatbelt her in place. You grab the bottle of medication to take with you to the hospital. You radio dispatch to see if the ALS ambulance can junction with you en route; however, you are informed that it is already on another call. You are 15 minutes from the nearest hospital. You note that the patient's level of consciousness has deteriorated.

6. What would you do for this patient now?

You should begin to assist ventilations with a bag-valve mask device. The respiratory distress is so severe that it is interfering with oxygenation of the brain. Supplemental oxygen via a nonrebreather mask is no longer sufficient. Begin to assist ventilations and move toward the ambulance.

You immediately begin to assist ventilations with a BVM connected to oxygen via a reservoir. You ask your partner to perform a quick head-to-toe exam. He reports that you are not getting much air in the lungs as evidenced by limited chest rise and fall and very diminished breath sounds.

7. What could you do to attempt to improve ventilation success?

You can attempt to perform several maneuvers. Since no trauma is suspected you should attempt to perform some neck extension as you would with a head tilt–chin lift maneuver. This should be supplemented by the placement of either an oral pharyngeal airway or a nasal pharyngeal airway.

You attempt to hyperextend the neck. No improvement is seen in ventilation success. You size and attempt to place an oral pharyngeal airway. You are unable to do so because the tongue is too swollen to allow it to pass. You size and then lubricate a nasal pharyngeal airway. You pass the device down the patient's right nare with no complications. The patient did not even respond to it being placed. You again attempt to ventilate and this time you see some improvement in chest rise and fall.

8. What should you do next?

You ask the patient if she has an Epi-pen and she shakes her head "no." Reassess the patient. You need to repeat your assessment of level of consciousness, airway, breathing, and circulatory status. It is possible that since the patient's respiratory status deteriorated so rapidly her circulatory system may also have been compromised. You need to assess for the onset of cardiac arrest to see if chest compressions will be necessary.

You ask your partner to repeat the primary survey as you continue to ventilate the patient. Your partner reports that she is now unresponsive to painful stimuli. Her airway is open with the nasal pharyngeal airway. She does have a palpable radial and carotid pulse, which is weak and rapid. She continues to have swelling of the face, lips, and soft tissues of the oral cavity. You are creating chest rise and fall during ventilation. He is able to auscultate some bilateral breath sounds with diffuse wheezing noted. Her abdomen is soft. The extremities are unremarkable except for the cyanosis that is noted.

9. What should your next action be?

You should begin transporting the patient to the ambulance. You have temporarily intervened by taking over her respiratory effort; however, the allergic reaction is still in progress. You should anticipate further swelling of the airway and continued deterioration of circulatory function. She simply needs more help than can be provided in the home or in an ambulance.

You transport the patient to the ambulance, where you secure her for transport. Your partner puts her on the automatic blood pressure machine before moving to the driver's seat of the ambulance. You begin transport to the nearest hospital, which is some 15 minutes away.

You are continuing to create chest rise and fall. You also note that her cyanosis is improving. The vital signs are: B/P 78/40, HR 158, SpO$_2$ of 89 percent, and you are ventilating her at a rate of 18 breaths per minute. You direct your partner to call in the report and to inform them of the medication she had been taking.

You are able to successfully ventilate her throughout the transport to the hospital. Upon arrival at the ED a team of physicians and nurses meets you. An anesthesiologist is waiting to take over the airway. After moving her to the ER bed, you see the physician pass a flexible tube into the patient's mouth. After much maneuvering he is able to pass a breathing tube called an endotracheal tube into her trachea. He is then able to ventilate her using the bag-valve device. Her color dramatically improves. During this time the staff initiate IV access and give several medications. You depart the room and debrief the call with your partner. You both prepare your truck for service.

PATIENT OUTCOME/PATHOPHYSIOLOGY

The patient did indeed suffer an anaphylactic reaction to her medication.

Amoxicillin (aka Amoxil) is an antibiotic from the penicillin class. It is utilized to fight numerous infective organisms and is usually prescribed in a capsule form. Caution should be taken with its administration as allergic reactions are possible.

She required the placement of an endotracheal tube for ventilation. Following IV placement she was administered IV epinephrine to improve her circulatory function. She was given IV Benadryl (antihistamine) to counteract the effects of the allergic immune response. Solu-Medrol (steroid) was administered to reduce the swelling of the soft tissues and pulmonary system. She was also given inhaled bronchodialators to improve her ventilatory status. She continued to improve and the following morning was removed from the respirator. She is going to make a complete recovery but now she must be aware of her newfound allergy to penicillin-class medications.

1. An anaphylactic reaction may be caused by which of the following?

   a. bee stings

   b. medications

   c. peanut butter

   d. all of the above

2. Partial airway obstructions caused by swelling of the tongue are best treated with which of the following?

   a. oral airway

   b. nasal pharyngeal airway

   c. head flexion

   d. bag-valve mask ventilation

3. Bluish discoloration of the skin caused by a lack of oxygen bound to hemoglobin is termed:

   a. mottling

   b. angioedema

   c. purpura

   d. cyanosis

4. In the absence of trauma the best technique for opening the airway of an adult patient is the:

   a. head flexion maneuver

   b. head tilt–chin lift maneuver

   c. Heimlich maneuver

   d. cricoid pressure maneuver

5. Difficulty swallowing may be caused by which of the following?

   a. stroke

   b. food bolus in the esophagus

   c. allergic reaction

   d. all of the above

6. Anaphylaxis may result in which of the following?

   a. respiratory compromise

   b. respiratory failure

   c. circulatory collapse

   d. death

   e. all of the above

7. Anaphylaxis may occur with the first exposure to an allergen.

    a. true

    b. false

8. Patients who are in severe respiratory distress and who have decreased levels of consciousness are best managed with which of the following oxygen-delivery systems?

    a. nasal cannula

    b. simple face mask

    c. nonrebreather mask

    d. bag-valve mask

9. The highest concentration of oxygen can be delivered by which of the following systems?

    a. nasal cannula

    b. simple face mask

    c. bag-valve mask

    d. bag-valve mask with an oxygen reservoir

10. Anaphylaxis is a load-and-go emergency.

    a. true

    b. false

22

MY HUSBAND WAS STUNG BY A BEE

Objectives

At the conclusion of this scenario, the participant will be able to:

1. Identify signs and symptoms of an allergic reaction.

2. Describe the difference between an allergic reaction and anaphylaxis.

3. Describe the appropriate indication and utilization of an epinephrine autoinjector.

SCENARIO

Your ambulance is dispatched to a local park following a "911" call from a cell phone. The caller reports that a bee, to which he is highly allergic, has stung her husband.

1. What concerns do you have regarding this information?

   You are very aware that bee stings may result in an allergic reaction. Bee venom, like many other insect venoms, may cause an immune response by the body. Foreign proteins from items such as bee venom, medications, foods, and chemicals may cause the body to release substances to combat them. If these substances are released too aggressively it may cause an allergic reaction that is very severe. We term this type of reaction "anaphylaxis." Anaphylaxis is so severe that it may lead to respiratory distress, respiratory failure, and circulatory collapse. If these go unmanaged then death may occur. The caller stated that her husband is allergic to bee stings; therefore, you should be prepared for a serious allergic reaction.

2. What should you do while en route to the call?

You and your partner should decide who will perform which functions during the call. You should also apply your BSI equipment, including gloves and eye protection. Also, because the caller stated that her husband is allergic to bee stings, you may wish to review your protocol regarding the assisted administration of epinephrine in the event that the patient has his own administration kit. These are commonly referred to as epi-pens. They contain a preset dose of epinephrine, which is injected by a spring-loaded needle. Some systems require that you contact medical control prior to administration. Others may allow you to administer the medication under standing orders. Review the protocol while en route to the call.

You arrive on location at the park. You are unable to see the caller, however. You slowly drive around until you hear a woman calling for you. You grab your equipment from the ambulance and quickly make your way to her location. There you see a man lying on the grass. He appears beet red and is covered in hives. He is having difficulty breathing as evidenced by his stridorous sounds.

3. What have you determined from this visual assessment?

This is a true emergency. This is a severe allergic reaction. You are able to identify many signs that indicate this. You see that the patient's skin is bright red in color. This usually indicates that the vessels below the skin are very dilated, allowing blood to be visible. You are able to identify hives, which are also characteristic of an allergic reaction. What concerns you most, however, is his difficulty with breathing. Stridorous respiratory sounds are indicative of constriction of the larger airway passages. This would represent the beginning of respiratory failure. This patient may stop breathing if you do not intervene promptly and appropriately.

You immediately direct your partner to apply oxygen at 15 Lpm via a nonrebreather mask and to assess vital signs. You approach the patient and begin your focused history and physical exam. You find that the patient is conscious but oriented to only his name. He does not know his location or the date. His airway is open but stridorous sounds are evident. You see that his lips and tongue are swollen. You are able to palpate a weak, rapid radial pulse. You ask the patient's wife if he has ever had this type of reaction before. She informs you that he has and that he even has medication for it. You ask him if he took the medication or if they have it with them. She tells you that he has not taken the medication and that it is in the car. You direct her to get the medication. Your partner reports the following vital signs: B/P 80/38, HR 148, RR 22, and an SpO_2 of 93 percent on oxygen.

4. What is your interpretation of this information?

Based upon your assessment you had determined that the patient was suffering from a severe allergic reaction. Now that you have the vital signs you know that the patient is also in shock from anaphylaxis.

You begin your head-to-toe survey while you are waiting for the patient's wife to return. The patient's LOC, airway, breathing, and circulation remain unchanged. The patient continues to have swollen lips and tongue. There is also noted swelling on the anterior aspect of the neck. The chest is covered in hives. Auscultation of breath sounds reveals diffuse wheezes and stridor in the upper airways. The abdomen is soft but reddened, with numerous hives as well. The extremities are reddened and also show hives. The patient no longer has a radial pulse but continues to have a rapid and weak brachial pulse.

5. What aspect of the patient's condition has changed?

    The patient has lost his radial pulse. This means that his blood pressure has dropped. His condition is worsening. You should expedite your move to the ambulance.

You and your partner place the patient on the stretcher and begin to move towards the ambulance. As you are loading the patient in the truck the wife runs to your side carrying a kit. It is labeled "EPI-PEN." You are aware that this is the medication utilized for severe allergic reaction. Your review of the protocols revealed that you are able to administer the epinephrine if the patient is unable to do so and evidence of anaphylaxis is noted.

6. What should you do now?

    You are at the ambulance. Secure the patient's stretcher and begin transport. There is nothing to be gained by delaying transport. This is a load-and-go situation.

7. Would you administer the medication on-scene?

    Since you are in the ambulance you should initiate transport. Epinephrine may be given en route if necessary. Severe anaphylaxis may require more than just the epinephrine available in this autoinjector. Expedite transport as soon as possible.

You secure the stretcher in the ambulance. You place the patient's wife on the bench seat and have her secure her safety belt. You begin emergency transport to the closest hospital, which is 10 minutes away. You reassess the primary survey and find that it is unchanged. You make the decision to utilize the epi-pen.

8. What do you need to ensure before you administer the medication?

    First, ensure that the medication belongs to the patient. Epinephrine is a powerful medication with many side effects. Do not administer, or even think of administering, the medication unless it belongs to him. If the medication does belong to the patient, you need to assess the medication as well. You will need to determine that the medication has not expired. You will also need to look at the medication to see if it is cloudy or discolored. This would indicate that the medication has gone bad. This could be very dangerous if administered. You will also want to read the instructions. There are several types of injectors that are available. Quickly familiarize yourself with the device before administration.

After examining the medication you determine that it does belong to the patient. It is also within its expiration time frame and the medicine looks clear without cloudiness or discoloration. You have also familiarized yourself with the administration technique. While you prepare the medication administration device you gather a SAMPLE history from the patient's wife. You find that his only allergy is bee venom. He takes no medications and only has this epi-pen prescribed. His past medical history reveals that he has had two previous anaphylactic reactions with the last being about 5 years ago. She states that they were just walking in the park and he had forgotten to take his medication along with him. She did not even think of it until you asked for it. He last ate some 4 hours ago. She did express that he started having problems so quickly that they didn't have time to react. You now prepare to administer the medication.

9. How does epinephrine help in the treatment of anaphylaxis?

Epinephrine (aka Adrenalin) is a sympathomimetic drug. This means that it will increase the pumping function of the heart and cause the airways to dilate. It also causes the arteries to constrict. These are desired responses when one is suffering from anaphylactic shock. This will cause an increase in blood pressure and also improve the ability of the patient to breathe.

Epinephrine has some side effects that may be seen and must be watched for. They include: increased heart rate, nausea/vomiting, increased anxiety, dizziness, headache, and chest pain. These are untoward side effects. You will need to continuously reassess the patient following epinephrine administration.

10. How do you administer epinephrine utilizing the autoinjector?
    a. Remove the cap from the injector.
    b. Place the tip of the auto injector against the patient's thigh midway between the knee and waist on the lateral aspect.
    c. Push the injector firmly into the surface of the skin.
    d. Continue to hold the injector in place until all medication is delivered. This may take from 10–15 seconds.
    e. Record the time of administration.
    f. Discard injector into Sharps Container.
    g. Reassess the patient for response.

Following the administration of the medication you call the hospital with a report, during which time you note that the patient begins to become more alert. You see that his skin appears less reddened. His stridor improves, as does his work of breathing. You reassess the patient and determine that he is improving. Your repeat vital signs are: B/P of 100/56, HR 140, RR 20, and SpO$_2$ of 99 percent on oxygen.

You continue to monitor the patient closely during transport. You arrive at the hospital where the patient is transferred to a bed in the emergency department. You give a verbal report and then complete the run form. You and your partner prepare the truck for your next run. You feel a sense of pride and relief as you realize that you did a good job, even though you had not touched an epi-pen since your initial EMT course.

PATIENT OUTCOME/PATHOPHYSIOLOGY

The patient continued to improve following your epinephrine administration. In the emergency department he was treated with Benadryl to combat the allergic reaction. He was also given a dose of Solu-Medrol (steroid) to reduce the inflammation in his lungs caused by his allergic reaction. He was monitored in the continuous observation unit for 23 hours before being discharged home. He immediately went to the pharmacy to refill his prescription for an epi-pen kit.

1. What initiates an allergic response by the body?

    a. anaphylaxis

    b. epinephrine

    c. allergens

    d. antibodies

2. What is the most severe type of allergic reaction called?

    a. hives

    b. purpura

    c. whelps

    d. anaphylaxis

3. Which of the following does epinephrine cause?

    a. bronchodilation

    b. arterial dilation

    c. decreased blood pressure

    d. all of the above

4. You may administer anyone's epinephrine to a patient who is truly in anaphylaxis.

    a. true

    b. false

5. Which of the following are reasons NOT to administer epinephrine?

    a. the medicine is clear in color

    b. it has a cloudy appearance

    c. it is within its expiration date

    d. all of the above

6. Patients who are allergic to insects who have been bitten but present with no signs of respiratory distress or circulatory compromise should be given epinephrine anyway.

    a. true

    b. false

7. Epi-pens should be administered at which of the following locations?

    a. lateral arm

    b. stomach

    c. lateral leg

    d. gluteus maximus of the buttocks

8. Epi-pens should be held in place for how long?
    a. it may be released immediately
    b. 5 seconds
    c. 10 seconds
    d. 30 seconds
    e. 1 minute

9. Patients with severe anaphylaxis who suffer from ineffective breathing are best treated with which of the following oxygen-delivery devices?
    a. nasal cannula
    b. nonrebreather mask
    c. bag-valve mask
    d. tracheostomy

10. Which of the following are signs of upper-airway constriction?
    a. wheezes
    b. stridor
    c. rales
    d. rhonchi

23

ATTEMPTED SUICIDE AT THE JAIL

Objectives

At the conclusion of this scenario, the participant will be able to:

1. Define the factors that increase the risk of suicide.

2. Describe the assessment and management of the suicidal patient.

3. Describe the management of soft tissue injuries with active bleeding.

SCENARIO

You are dispatched to the county jail where police officers have brought in a 45-year-old female who tried to kill herself. Apparently, she cut her wrists with her soon-to-be ex-husband's hunting knife.

1. Based on the limited information provided, are there any clues as to why this woman has attempted to harm herself?

   Did you note the "soon-to-be ex-husband" comment? Obviously this woman is having marital problems, which could certainly explain her actions. Divorce is a very common factor in many suicides. Other precursors to suicide include alcoholism, depression, the loss of a job, financial difficulties, and other psychiatric disturbances such as schizophrenia.

   You and your partner are escorted into the building by the jailor. As you approach the patient, who appears very depressed, you see that both of her wrists are wrapped with towels, which have spots of dark red, dried blood on them.

2. How will you approach this patient initially, considering her present condition?

Very carefully! This patient has not only threatened suicide, she has made an attempt. You also do not know if she also assaulted her husband or another, causing her incarceration. Though she may appear reserved right now, any attempt to make contact (verbal or physical) with her could cause her to become violent. Ensure that at least one police officer remains in the room with you as you assess her.

You sit in a chair near the patient and ask her what her name is. After a brief delay, she replies "Sharon." You ask her what happened and she states that she is tired of being made a fool of by her husband, who she claims is having an affair. She then clenches her fists and begins to cry.

3. Are there any personal safety concerns at this point?

   Most definitely! Emotionally disturbed patients, as previously mentioned, can become extremely violent without warning; however, this patient is displaying a classic warning sign of potential violence: clenched fists. In addition, just because she is crying does not mean that she is "letting it all out." It could indicate a potential outburst of anger that is building within her. You must be prepared to retreat to a place of safety if needed.

4. What will be your approach to assessing and managing her injuries?

   At this point, it is too premature to attempt to expose this patient's injuries. Since her wounds do not appear to be bleeding uncontrollably, you should focus more on attempting to calm the patient and gain her trust, which may take some time and patience on your part.

After talking to the patient for approximately 7–10 minutes, she consents to you looking at her injuries. You remove the towels from her wrists and note the presence of several lacerations, approximately 1–2 inches in length with minimal bleeding. You assess sensation and circulation distal to the injuries. As you begin to cover the wounds with sterile dressings, you ask her if she is injured anywhere else. She says that those are her only injuries. Your partner begins to place a blood pressure cuff on the patient's arm to obtain baseline vital signs.

5. How might the patient respond to your partner's actions?

   Violence! Nothing should be done to this patient without her permission, and although this is true with all patients, consent prior to treatment with this particular patient is even more important. Just because she allowed you to cover her wounds does not imply consent to full assessment and management. Remember, emotionally disturbed patients can be calm and cooperative one minute and violent the next. You want to minimize this risk as much as possible.

After obtaining baseline vital signs, which were stable, you proceed into the SAMPLE history. She denies allergies and has a past medical history of depression, for which she takes Prozac. She states that she has not eaten in 2 days and that subsequent to an argument with her husband, she cut herself. At this point, you ask her if she would allow you to take her to the hospital for further evaluation. She states "Yeah, right . . . a psycho farm, huh?"

6. What aspects of the SAMPLE history are consistent with her present situation and what additional questions should you ask?

Clearly, with the history of depression, she is in a high-risk group for suicide, which she has proven. It is very common for severely depressed patients to go for days without eating. Prozac is an antidepressant medication. In addition to the questions already asked during the SAMPLE history, it would be appropriate to ask her when she last took her medication as well as whether or not she attempted an overdose.

7. How should you respond to the statement that the patient made after you asked to transport her to the hospital?

With the problems that this patient is experiencing, it is not unreasonable for her to assume that you are going to transport her to a psychiatric facility. You must assure the patient that as an EMT, your job is to transport all patients to the emergency department, where a physician will evaluate them. Additional treatment beyond that will be determined by a more detailed assessment in the emergency department.

The patient consents to transport. You tell her that you will take her to the facility of her choice. She states that she has no money or insurance and wishes to go to the county hospital. You allow her to walk to the ambulance and begin transport to the hospital, which is approximately 15 miles away.

8. Are there any special considerations during transport?

You must continually monitor the patient with regards to both her physical and emotional status. If you feel threatened or think that the patient may become uncooperative en route (you should be prepared for this), you may want to request that a police officer accompany you in the back of the ambulance. Since the patient is in custody this may occur anyway. If the patient indeed becomes violent, not only will you have additional help in the ambulance, but you will have a witness who will concur with the need to restrain the patient should it become necessary.

After a 20-minute transport, you deliver the patient to the hospital without incident. You give report to the attending physician and return your ambulance to service.

PATIENT OUTCOME/PATHOPHYSIOLOGY

The patient was briefly assessed in the emergency department. After her wounds were cleaned and sutured, she was admitted to the psychiatric ward of the hospital for temporary care until transport to a definitive care psychiatric facility could be arranged.

Severe clinical depression is a significant risk factor for suicide. Other risk factors include alcoholism, depression, and those who are single, widowed, or divorced. Patients who have a detailed suicide plan (taking a series of actions rather than a single impulsive act) are also at a greater risk of suicide. While people with multiple unsuccessful suicide attempts are often regarded as "looking for attention," those with prior attempts are statistically more likely to actually commit suicide. Suicide represents the patient's perceived resolution to the problem. They feel that the problem will resolve if they are no longer a part of it. Indeed it resolves their problems, but causes many more problems for a great number of people (family, friends, and EMTs).

EVALUATION

1. A patient who is threatening suicide but has not attempted it should be managed by:
   a. transporting to a psychiatric facility based upon the orders of the police
   b. restraining the patient and transporting to the hospital with police escort
   c. carefully assessing the patient and planning to spend extra time with him
   d. treating the patient as any other patient, avoiding questions specific to suicide

2. Initial management for a patient who has cut his wrists, is actively bleeding, and threatening to hit you includes:
   a. making immediate attempts to control the bleeding
   b. protecting yourself by approaching the patient carefully
   c. having the police restrain the patient so you can control the bleeding
   d. not making contact with the patient until the police have arrived

3. Risk factors for suicide include all of the following EXCEPT:
   a. depression
   b. a brief illness
   c. schizophrenia
   d. loss of a loved one

4. Your primary concern in managing a patient who has attempted suicide is:
   a. whether the patient has a history of suicide
   b. to determine why the patient tried to kill himself
   c. whether or not the patient will try to harm you
   d. to determine what medications the patient is taking

5. Management of a soft tissue injury in an emotionally disturbed patient includes:
   a. not managing the injury as the patient may become violent
   b. assessing sensation and circulation distal to the injury
   c. restraining the patient prior to managing the injury
   d. foregoing management if the patient remains calm

6. The police have arrived on the scene of an attempted suicide. Evidently, a young male shot himself in the head with a .22 caliber handgun. As your unit arrives at the scene, your primary concern should be to:

    a. provide immediate care to the patient
    b. preserve any potential evidence
    c. ensure that the gun has been secured
    d. call for additional police officers

7. A common route that females will take in a suicide attempt includes:

    a. hanging themselves
    b. self-inflicted gunshot wounds
    c. running their car into a tree
    d. overdosing on medications

8. A common medication used for the treatment of depression is:

    a. digoxin
    b. nitroglycerin
    c. Prozac
    d. ibuprofen

9. Factors that indicate potential violence in the psychiatric patient include:

    a. the size of the patient
    b. clenching of the fists
    c. the age and sex of the patient
    d. a family history of violence

10. Which of the following presents the least risk of a successful suicide attempt?

    a. history of alcoholism
    b. significant depression
    c. prior suicide attempts
    d. the patient's age

24

MY STOMACH HURTS

Objectives

At the conclusion of this scenario, the participant will be able to:

1. Discuss causes of lower-quadrant abdominal pain.

2. List signs and symptoms of intra-abdominal bleeding.

3. Identify treatment options for patients suffering from ectopic pregnancies.

SCENARIO

Your ambulance has been dispatched to the gym of a local high school. The caller reports that they have an 18-year-old girl who collapsed to the ground, stating that her stomach hurts. She is reported as conscious and writhing in pain. Your estimated time of arrival is 5 minutes.

1. What are your thoughts concerning this dispatch information?

   Your dispatch has answered your first concern. At this time, at least, the patient is conscious; therefore, CPR is likely not in progress. Your next thoughts turn to the cause of a young person collapsing to the ground from abdominal pain. There are many causes of severe abdominal pain. Fortunately, a young person typically only suffers from a few of these major causes. Some examples of causes include: appendicitis, torsion of bowel, ovarian cyst, fallopian tubal pregnancy, and severe gas pain, just to name a few.

   You arrive at the high school where administration directs you into the gym area. The first thing you note is a large group of students standing not far from the patient who is lying on the floor. There are several teachers and coaches who are next to the victim.

2. What should your next action be?

Your first action should be scene control. Have administration move the students away from the immediate area. This will decrease patient apprehension regarding her peer's unnecessary attendance. Also, direct nonessential teachers and coaches to move further away from the patient so you can begin your assessment and treatment. Remember, however, that someone with the school should have a file containing the patient's pertinent medical history and may also be helpful in describing the events that occurred. Be very tactful when moving nonessential personnel aside.

Also remember that some teenagers and children will not share information that could somehow get back to their parents. Providing space and ensuring that the information you gain will remain confidential may increase the likeliness that the patient will share personal information with you.

After clearing the area of nonessential personnel you finally make patient contact. You immediately ascertain if the patient fell or suffered any other type of trauma. You are informed that no fall or injury was sustained. She immediately began to cry out in pain and sat down on the floor. You begin assessing the LOC, airway, breathing, and circulation status of the patient. You note that she is awake and crying in pain. Her airway is open and patent but she is breathing somewhat fast. Palpation of her pulse reveals that she has no radial pulse but does have a weak and rapid brachial pulse. You also note that her skin feels clammy and her color is somewhat pale.

3. Is this an emergency situation? What are your thoughts regarding the information you found during your primary survey?

Absolutely. This patient has several signs and symptoms of shock. She has pale, clammy skin along with rapid heart rate, rapid breathing, and no palpable radial pulse. This in conjunction with abdominal pain is a serious condition.

You immediately direct your partner to place the patient on oxygen at 15 Lpm with a nonrebreather mask and then to perform a set of vital signs as you begin your focused history and physical exam. You ask the patient what happened and how she feels now. She informs you that she felt fine this morning and was just participating in the game of dodge ball when she suddenly was overcome with pain; she points to her right lower-quadrant area. She said it felt like something was tearing inside of her.

4. What is the most common cause of right lower-quadrant (RLQ) abdominal pain in young persons? What other structures found in this area should also be considered as possible causes?

The most common cause of RLQ abdominal pain is appendicitis. However, the appendix generally becomes inflamed for several hours to days before it causes rupture. Most patients complain of low-grade fever, nausea, and an onset of pain, which gradually intensifies. In female patients you must also consider inflammation or injury to female anatomy. You should consider conditions such as an ovarian cyst or pelvic inflammatory disease as potential causes. In women of childbearing age (10–60 years of age) you should always consider ectopic pregnancy (fetus implanted and growing anywhere other than the uterus) as a po-

tential cause. The problem with ectopic pregnancies is that as the fetus continues to grow and expand in size, it will eventually cause injury to surrounding structures if not implanted within the uterus. For example, if implantation occurs within the fallopian tube or oviduct it will eventually tear, causing severe pain and bleeding within the pelvic region. If the implantation occurs outside of the female reproductive structures, as in the case of a fertilized egg exiting the ovaries and escaping through the finger-like structures of the fallopian tube opening, it may begin to develop in the pelvic cavity. We call these "extrauterine pregnancies." Eventually they may cause severe pain and bleeding to surrounding structures.

You begin to gather information regarding the onset, provocation, quality, radiation, severity, and time (O, P, Q, R, S, and T) of her pain. The patient now describes the pain as a constant burning sensation that hurts across the lower portion of her abdomen. She rates it as a 10 on a 1–10 scale. You immediately place the patient in a supine position and place one of your response bags under her legs as you continue your assessment. Your partner reports the following vital signs: B/P of 88/40, HR 130, RR 24, pupils are equal and reactive to light, and the patient has an SpO$_2$ reading of 99 percent on oxygen. You ask your partner to prepare the stretcher as you begin your physical assessment. Your primary survey remains unchanged. Her breath sounds are clear and equal bilaterally. The patient denies nausea. Palpation of her abdomen reveals severe, constant pain that is now in all of the lower abdomen. Her abdomen is semi-firm to palpation and she is guarding it during your palpation. Her pelvis is stable with no reports of any vaginal discharge. Her extremities are unremarkable except for her decreased peripheral perfusion.

5. What is the significance of your finding during the abdominal exam?

   Abdominal pain is difficult to assess. Oftentimes patients describe pain as either sharp, dull, or tearing. Tearing is generally just that—a sensation of a visceral structures being ripped. Examples include the tearing of an aorta during dissection and the tearing of a fallopian tube during ectopic pregnancy. Sharp pain is often related to colic like gas pain or acute inflammation as in the case of diverticulitis. Dull pain may also be caused by pressure-like situations such as constipation or gas but may also occur with bleeding within the abdominal cavity. Pain that is made worse with palpation may also indicate bleeding within the abdominal cavity.

You and your partner place the girl on the stretcher, keeping her in a shock position. Oxygen is also continued. You are given her medical records, which are reported as containing only information regarding her immunizations. You immediately begin transporting her to your waiting ambulance.

6. What is the next portion of your assessment that you may perfom en route to the ambulance?

   You need to perform a SAMPLE history. This may provide valuable information about the cause of her pain.

   NOTE: Always ask about "last menstrual cycle" in patients of childbearing age. Remember this by adding it with the "L" portion of the assessment.

You begin to ascertain the information regarding the SAMPLE history. Her symptoms remain as previously described. She states that her only allergy is to Tetracycline (an antibiotic). She takes no medications but she has approached her mother about beginning "the pill." She denies any past medical history. Her last meal was breakfast about 3 hours ago. You also ask her about her last menstrual cycle and whether or not there is any chance that she might be pregnant. She responds, "No way. I've only had sex twice and we have been very careful." She also states that her cycles are not always the same and that she should start very soon. The events regarding the situation also remain unchanged.

7. What are your thoughts regarding the information gained during your SAMPLE history?

A majority of the SAMPLE history is benign. However, the information gained during assessment for possible pregnancy is invaluable. Teenagers sometimes believe that they can't get pregnant during their first couple of sexual experiences. This is most definitely wrong. You can get pregnant the very first time. She also describes her cycle as being somewhat irregular. This is very common. Typically the female menstrual cycle operates around a 28-day period with the menses portion of the cycle lasting from 3–5 days. It is also possible for someone to be pregnant and still have some remnant of menses following egg implantation. Remember: A female patient of childbearing age who complains of abdominal pain is pregnant until proven otherwise by a physician.

NOTE: "The pill" is a common term utilized for birth control (BC) medications. These are hormones that alter the ability for an egg to implant itself if fertilized. Despite high success rates in preventing pregnancy, the only 100 percent effective technique is abstinence. Women can and do get pregnant while on birth control medications. Because of this they are also subject to complications of pregnancy such as ectopic pregnancy.

You place the patient in the ambulance and secure her for transport. You begin emergency transport to the area hospital some 7 minutes away. You continue oxygen therapy and reassess vital signs, which are essentially unchanged. You radio a report to the emergency department detailing your findings and intervention. You also inform them that you are suspicious of an "ectopic pregnancy."

You deliver the patient to the emergency department where a team of physicians, surgeons, and nursing personnel are awaiting your arrival. You complete your report and prepare to return to service.

PATIENT OUTCOME/PATHOPHYSIOLOGY

Your patient was assessed in the emergency department by a team of physicians and surgeons. An ultrasound of the pelvis and lower abdomen was performed. Blood was noted in the lower abdomen and pelvic region. They also noted that the fallopian tube was torn, confirming your suspicion of a tubular ectopic pregnancy. She was immediately taken to the operating room where she received 4 units of blood and underwent surgical repair of her right fallopian region. She was hospitalized for 6 days before being discharged home. A full recovery is expected.

EVALUATION

1. Where should normal fertilized egg implantation occur?
   a. ovaries
   b. fallopian tubes
   c. uterus
   d. cervix

2. What is the length of the typical menstrual cycle?
   a. 24 days
   b. 28 days
   c. 1 month
   d. 6 weeks

3. What is the most common cause of RLQ abdominal pain in young people?
   a. colic
   b. diverticulitis
   c. appendicitis
   d. ovarian cyst

4. What is the cause of shock in a patient suffering from a ruptured fallopian ectopic pregnancy?
   a. pain
   b. blood loss
   c. psychogenic shock
   d. septic shock

5. Which of the following are signs of intra-abdominal bleeding?
   a. pain
   b. guarding of the abdomen
   c. rapid heart rate
   d. rapid breathing
   e. all of the above

6. A female patient of childbearing age who complains of abdominal pain should be considered pregnant until proven otherwise by a physician.
   a. true
   b. false

7. "The pill" typically refers to which of the following medications?
   a. ecstasy
   b. birth control medication

c. Retinae

d. LSD

8. Woman cannot get pregnant from their first sexual experience.

   a. true

   b. false

9. Which technique would increase the likelihood that a teenager would share personal information with you?

   a. provide an area free from peers and parents

   b. ensure that the information will remain confidential

   c. display a nonjudgmental attitude

   d. all of the above

10. Treatment of an ectopic pregnancy includes which of the following?

   a. administration of fluid by mouth to combat shock

   b. applying direct pressure to the lower abdominal quadrant that hurts

   c. transportation to a hospital that can provide immediate surgery

   d. being prepared for an imminent delivery

25

I'M HAVING A BABY

Objectives

At the conclusion of this scenario, the participant will be able to:

1. Discuss the signs of imminent childbirth.

2. List questions that should be asked during imminent deliveries.

3. Discuss treatment of complications that may occur during childbirth.

SCENARIO

Your ambulance is dispatched to a residence 20 minutes out in the country. Dispatch reports that the caller states that she is having a baby.

1. What are your considerations regarding this dispatch information?

   Simply put: imminent delivery. You must be prepared, upon arrival, to either participate in the immediate delivery of a newborn or to manage the mother and infant of a delivery that has already occurred.

2. What preparations should you make while en route to the call?

   You should inquire about further information from the dispatcher. If the information appears as though delivery is imminent then you may need to request back-up personnel, especially if the delivery is premature or if complications have arisen. Personal protective equipment should be gathered to include protective eyewear and gloves at minimum. A gown will also be necessary. Along with normal response bags you will need to grab your emergency obstetric (OB) kit to take to the patient's side.

131

No further information was available from the dispatcher. They stated when they attempted to call back to the residence that no one answered the phone. Upon arrival at the residence you ensure scene safety as you approach the home. You immediately hear someone crying inside the home. After knocking you are told to enter by a woman's voice. Again ensuring your own and your partner's safety, you enter the home. As you enter the living area of the home you see a female, approximately 25 years old, lying on the sofa. She is conscious and is crying. She says, "Please help me."

3. What information have you learned from this brief encounter?

    You have gained valuable information from the primary survey of this patient. She is conscious and appears alert. She is able to speak and may be oriented, which is the beginning of your initial assessment. She has also given a form of consent by asking for your help. You will now need to gain the remainder of your focused history and physical exam.

    The patient is obviously pregnant by her apparent gravid uterus. You ask her what is wrong and why she is crying. She explains that her water broke suddenly about 25 minutes ago and that she is about 5 weeks early.

4. How long does the normal pregnancy last? What is the significance of the above information?

    The normal pregnancy lasts 40 weeks. Most laypersons believe that a pregnancy lasts only 9 months. The significance of this information is that the patient states she is 5 weeks early. This would indicate that the fetus is only 35 weeks along in its development. A newborn delivered at 35 weeks will be smaller than an infant born at term. You would also expect that the lungs will not be as mature nor will its heart regulatory ability be as developed as that of a term infant. You must be ready to handle this newborn should delivery occur.

5. What should your next step be in the assessment of this woman?

    You should immediately assess for the presence of an imminent delivery situation. Perform a focused physical assessment regarding the chance of her delivering. You may ask questions that are pertinent to her labor as you assess for vaginal bulging, crowning, or abnormal presentation of the fetus.

    You immediately begin a focused assessment regarding the likelihood of an imminent delivery. You again ask her about her water breaking. You inquire as to the amount and its color. You also ask about prenatal care, specifically if any abnormalities were found during her pregnancy. You also explain that you need to visually assess her pelvic region to see if she is going to have this baby now.

6. What is the significance of her "water breaking" and its appearance?

    Laypersons utilize the term "bag of water" to describe the amniotic sac that surrounds the newborn during uterine development. When they say that "my water broke" they are actually referring to the rupture of the amniotic sac. Amniotic fluid is then leaked from the vagina via the cervical opening. It is important to note the color of the amniotic fluid. For example, if the fluid is foul colored and/or foul smelling it may indicate that there was actually an infection of the fluid while surrounding the baby. If the fluid contains green- or brown-colored material it may indicate the presence of "meconium." Meconium is actually the contents of the baby's lower gastrointestinal tract. Meconium should not be released from the baby while it remains in the uterus. When the baby releases meconium while in utero it typically indicates that the baby had severe distress that caused this to occur. Meconium floating in the amniotic fluid may be taken into the baby's lungs, causing severe respiratory complications upon delivery and the days following delivery.

7. Why would you ask her about her pregnancy and if she had any complications?

You are trying to determine if her physician or midwife noted any complications. Complications such as growth retardation, fluid on the brain, spinal bifida, or any other structural abnormalities may lead to a complication during or following delivery. An excellent mnemonic to remember is the "4 M's":

- Maturation—How far along is the fetus? When is delivery supposed to occur?
- Meconium—Was there any meconium present in the amniotic fluid?
- Multiples—Is there any possibility that she may be pregnant with more than one child?
- Medications—What medications has she taken? Prescribed, over-the-counter, or herbal medications should all be determined.

You determine that her amniotic fluid was clear. She is 35 weeks along in her first pregnancy, as determined by dates and by ultrasound. There have been no complications during her pregnancy. The only medication that she has taken during her pregnancy is prenatal vitamins (PNV). She states that she felt the urge to push a short time ago and that she did. She says that she has been having contractions off and on all afternoon but now they are about 5 minutes apart and lasting 30–40 seconds. You visually assess her vaginal region.

8. Why is it important to know how often and how long contractions are?

Women who are pregnant for the first time usually take longer to deliver a baby. The average is usually 16–18 hours. Contraction length and regularity are essential. The shorter the time between contractions the shorter the time to delivery. Women who are contracting between 3–5 minutes apart are approaching the time of delivery.

NOTE: Prenatal vitamins (PNVs) are supplements prescribed to pregnant women to assist in ensuring they get an adequate daily amount of necessary vitamins and minerals to meet the demands of their own body, as well as the needs of the unborn child.

Upon visual assessment of the vagina you see that a cord-like item is protruding from the vagina. You witness no crowning or presenting fetal parts. She states that she needs to push.

9. What is the significance of this presentation?

This is a true emergency. The cord-like structure is the umbilical cord. The umbilical cord is the "lifeline" of the unborn infant and the infant as it is being delivered. We term this situation a "prolapsed cord," meaning that it has delivered before the baby. The significance being that as the child enters the birth canal it will compress its own lifeline. Immediate action *must be taken to prevent the entry of the infant into the birth canal or to ensure that it doesn't compress its own cord if already in the canal. You will do this manually by inserting a gloved hand inside the vagina and applying pressure to the presenting part of the baby (use caution if face is presenting) to prevent further delivery. This must be maintained until such time that the mother is delivered to the hospital and someone is ready to take your place. Delivery should be performed by caesarean section.*

10. Should you allow the patient to push?

NO! If the mother continues to push during contractions she will further engage the infant in the birth canal. This may completely compress the umbilical cord causing the oxygenated blood supply of the baby to be cut off. This may lead to the death of the infant before delivery.

You instruct the patient not to push. You explain to the woman the situation that has occurred. You inform her of the treatment you must immediately employ and why. You insert your gloved hand inside the vagina. You are able to feel what you believe is the baby's head at the cervical opening. You begin to apply pressure on the baby's head to prevent further delivery. You are also careful not to compress the umbilical cord with your hand. You then feel the cord that is protruding and you are able to feel it pulsate. You instruct your partner to immediately place the patient on oxygen at 15 Lpm via a nonrebreather mask and to place a moistened 4 × 4 gauze pad over the exposed umbilical cord.

11. What are your thoughts regarding transport at this time?

Immediate transport is warranted. With a 20-minute transport evident you may wish to consider aeromedical transport if available. A helicopter would be very appropriate for this situation. If not available, you will need to transport this patient to the closest facility that can perform a c-section. If you and your partner will be transporting this patient, there are some things to consider:

- *It will be difficult for you and your partner to lower and raise the stretcher with you preventing further fetal delivery. Enlist neighbors or other EMS/law enforcement personnel for assistance.*
- *Utilize your left hand to insert in the vagina if you will be transporting in a Type II (van style) ambulance or a Type I/III ambulance, which has the stretcher mounted against the wall. Otherwise you will have no place to sit during transport.*

12. Why should you place a moistened 4 × 4 guaze on the exposed umbilical cord?

By placing a moistened 4 × 4 guaze on the exposed umbilical cord you will prevent it from drying due to exposure to room air. As the umbilical cord dries it will cause the cord to shrink in girth. This will cause contraction of the umbilical arteries and veins, which would also cause obstruction of blood flow to the infant.

You have decided to call for a medical helicopter to aid in transport. Their ETA is 12 minutes. The Sheriff's office has dispatched deputies to set up a landing zone. You direct your partner to perform vital signs on the mother. B/P is 138/62, HR is 110, RR is 20, and she has an SpO_2 of 100 percent on oxygen. You gather a SAMPLE history while waiting for the aircraft. The mother denies medication allergies and is again insisting that the only medication she takes is PNV. She has no past medical history and this is her only pregnancy. She last ate about 3 hours ago. She asks you to call her husband so he can be at the hospital and you direct your partner to perform that task.

The helicopter arrives landing in a field adjacent to the woman's home. The flight crew arrives and you give a detailed report as to what has transpired up to this point. They direct you to continue therapy as they assist in placing the patient on a stretcher and begin transport to the aircraft. There you are relieved by a flight crewmember who, following the removal of your hand, inserts her gloved hand to prevent further delivery of the infant. Shortly thereafter, the aircraft departs the scene for its 7-minute flight to County General. You and your partner gather your equipment, lock the home, and depart the scene. En route back to the station you begin writing your report.

PATIENT OUTCOME/PATHOPHYSIOLOGY

The mother was transported to County General by helicopter. The flight crew requested that an OB physician be waiting upon their arrival. Seven minutes after departure the mother was taken into the emergency department where she was seen by an obstetrician. She was immediately moved to an operating room where an emergency c-section was performed. The mother did well following the operation. The newborn was placed in a neonatal intensive care unit where he remains on a breathing machine. The physician does state that the prognosis for the infant is excellent and a full recovery is expected.

EVALUATION

1. What is the average length of a normal pregnancy?
   a. 35 weeks
   b. 36 weeks
   c. 38 weeks
   d. 40 weeks

2. What is the average length of labor time for a woman delivering her first child?
   a. 24 hours
   b. 16 hours
   c. 12 hours
   d. 10 hours

3. Which assessment findings indicate the greatest chance of imminent delivery?
   a. contractions lasting 45 seconds that are 10 minutes apart
   b. contractions lasting 48 seconds that are 8 minutes apart
   c. contractions lasting 48 seconds that are 5 minutes apart
   d. contractions lasting 50 seconds that are 3 minutes apart

4. Release of fecal matter into the amniotic fluid by the fetus is termed:

   a. phlegm
   b. surfactant
   c. fundus
   d. meconium

5. Premature infants are at risk for which of the following?

   a. respiratory complications
   b. heat regulation complications
   c. sugar maintenance complications
   d. all of the above

6. Which of the following are part of the "4 M's" of assessment?

   a. maturation
   b. materials
   c. muscle rigidity
   d. motion in the abdomen

7. When an umbilical cord has prolapsed it is necessary to immediately clamp the cord so that delivery can continue.

   a. true
   b. false

8. The fetus receives oxygenated blood from the umbilical cord via which of the following structures?

   a. amniotic sac
   b. fundus
   c. placenta
   d. spleen

9. Following delivery of a baby it generally takes how long to deliver the placenta?

   a. 5–10 minutes
   b. 15–20 minutes
   c. 30–40 minutes
   d. greater than 40 minutes

10. If a mother displays signs of supine hypotension syndrome you should immediately:

    a. place the mother on her left side
    b. sit her in an upright position
    c. lay her flat and elevate the legs
    d. give her something to drink

26

PREGNANT AND BLEEDING

Objectives

At the conclusion of this scenario, the participant will be able to:

1. List two causes of bleeding in the third trimester of pregnancy.

2. List the steps of patient care for patients with vaginal bleeding.

3. Describe the assessment of the pregnant patient.

SCENARIO

Your EMS unit is dispatched to a residence about 10 miles outside the city. The dispatcher informs you that the caller, who is the patient, had a sudden onset of vaginal bleeding. The patient states she is 31 weeks along in her first pregnancy. She is alone and scared.

1. What are your thoughts pertaining to the dispatch information?

   Vaginal bleeding can lead to a hypovolemic shock condition in the pregnant patient. It is also a type of bleeding that cannot be controlled. There are no prearrival dispatcher instructions that can slow or stop the bleeding. As maternal bleeding continues blood will also be diverted from the baby. This patient is also very early in her pregnancy (31 weeks). A normal pregnancy lasts 40 weeks, actually longer than the 9 months most laypersons believe. Delivery at this time would produce a small, premature infant at risk for many preterm complications.

   Ensure that you take an obstetrical (OB) kit with you into the home along with your other response kits. Imminent delivery is a possibility.

   You arrive on scene. You and your partner approach the home carrying your first-in bag and an OB kit. After knocking on the door you hear a female voice telling you to come in because she can't come to the door. You are cautious as you enter the home, ensuring your own and your partner's safety. You find a female patient, in her mid-20s, lying supine on the couch. She is slightly pale in color and you note blood on her dress and the couch cushion underneath her. She tells you that she isn't due for another 2½ months. She states that everything was fine and then suddenly, about half an hour ago, she just started bleeding. She felt too weak to drive to the ER.

2. What are your priorities at this time?

    Put on your personal protective equipment (PPE), which should include gloves and eye protection at a minimum. Active hemorrhage may lead to a source of exposure for you and your partner.

    Begin your initial assessment. If the patient is able to talk full sentences without catching her breath and without abnormal sounds or effort, you know that her airway is open and that she is breathing adequately. The patient is bleeding. Check circulation and pulses. Begin by comparing her central pulse (carotid) to her distal pulse (radial). Carotid pulses without radial pulses being present would indicate a severe shock condition. This would imply that blood is being "shunted" or its distribution is being limited to the extremities.

3. How much blood do you estimate that she has lost?

    Healthcare personnel in general are inaccurate at estimating blood loss. Small amounts of blood may appear substantial when they are on a kitchen floor. Large amounts of blood may appear small when they are contained within a car seat or, as in this case, a couch cushion. Assume that a substantial amount of blood has been lost.

4. Should you assess Mom first or immediately begin assessing the unborn child?

    The initial management of obstetrical emergencies always begins with assessment and care of the mother. The unborn child (fetus) is dependent upon its mother for the delivery of adequate amounts of oxygen and nutrients via the placenta. The placenta is dependent upon the mother to have adequate circulation to deliver the oxygen and nutrients. The secondary assessment will include a visual assessment of the vagina and perineal area. The presence and quantity of vaginal discharge or bleeding will be observed. You will also look for crowning of the baby, presentation of a baby's part other than the head, or bulging of the vagina. Each of these would indicate imminent delivery.

    You complete your patient assessment and begin providing care as you prepare for patient transport.

    NOTE: Prenatal vitamins are a commonly prescribed supplement during the course of a pregnancy. Many women alter their diets during pregnancy due to common bouts of upset stomach and gastric complaints. The name of the vitamins may be abbreviated on the bottle as "PNV."

Your assessment reveals that the mother's airway is open and that she is breathing well. You find that her pulses are weak and thready. Her heart rate is 130 beats/minute. Her skin color is pale and she is sweating on her forehead and upper lip. She asks for a drink of water. Her lung sounds are clear. Assessment of her abdomen reveals a palpable, pregnant uterus (fundus). Visual exam of her vagina and perineal area demonstrate no crowning or vaginal bulging. However, you do note a steady "ooze" of darkened blood coming from the vaginal opening. Vital signs are: B/P 100/58, HR 130, RR 22. The remainder of her patient assessment is unremarkable. When gathering your SAMPLE history information you find that she denies any allergies to medications. She states that she is taking daily prenatal vitamins. She has no significant PMH (Past Medical History). She admits to eating breakfast about 2 hours ago. She informs you that her OB physician is Dr. Speck.

5. What do you think is the major complication based on the patient assessment?

Shock! Rapid (HR 130), weak, and thready pulses are all signs of shock caused by hypovolemia. Thirst is also a symptom of shock. Made worse is the fact that we cannot stop this type of blood loss. Another complication is that the mother's shock is also affecting the unborn child. You have no way of monitoring the fetal response to Mom's shock state.
    Do not give the mother anything to drink as it may lead to nausea and vomiting.

6. What interventions would you perform initially?

Begin oxygen administration. Use a nonrebreather (NRB) mask at 15 Lpm. Shock treatment also includes positioning the patient in a supine position and keeping her warm by covering her with a sheet or blanket. You may even elevate her legs somewhat to improve return of blood flow from the lower extremities. Place the patient on the stretcher and prepare for immediate transport. This is a true emergency.

Oxygen is applied to the patient at 15 Lpm with an NRB mask. The patient is moved to the stretcher. Her legs are elevated and she is covered with a blanket.

7. What changes in shock treatment position should be made for pregnant patients?

Pregnant patients who are past their 20th week of pregnancy should never lay flat on their backs. They should be tilted to the left side at least 30 degrees. As the fetus increases in size and weight within the uterus it may cause compression of the mother's inferior vena cava (the largest vein in the lower half of the body). The uterus will act like a weight, causing blood return from the lower half of the body to "dam-up." This causes a decrease in blood return to the mother's heart, which then leads to a decrease in outflow of blood from the mother's heart. This may actually cause, in some cases, or worsen shock in pregnant patients.
    You place the patient in a left lateral recumbent position supported by pillows or folded blankets.

8. How is bleeding from the vagina controlled?

It can't be. Never place anything inside the vagina to stop or slow bleeding. Instead, place an item to catch what is coming out to determine if the rate of bleeding slows or increases. Place a vaginal pad over the vagina. If one is not available an ABD pad or trauma dressing may be used.
    If the pad becomes saturated, simply remove it and replace it with another. Pads that have been removed should be saved and transported with the patient to the hospital. They will be used to estimate how much blood has been lost.

You have placed the patient in the ambulance and have initiated emergent transport to the hospital. Early notification is given to the hospital so it can be prepared to handle this obstetrical emergency. Many hospitals may have to call in additional personnel to handle this emergency. During your transport you are cautious as you continue to reevaluate your patient's response. You frequently examine the vaginal pad to see if bleeding remains the same or has changed for better or worse.

During the transport to the hospital you note that the mother continues to remain awake and alert. You see that her color has also improved somewhat as well. She is no longer diaphoretic. She continues to ask if she can have some water. She states she is also very scared. "I don't want to lose my baby!" You continue to calm her and reassure her that everything that can be done is being done. You reassess her vital signs and they are noted to be: B/P 108/64, HR 122, RR 20.

You arrive safely at the hospital where the ER physician, nurses, and Dr. Speck are waiting to assume care for the patient. You complete your report as your partner prepares the ambulance for the next emergency.

PATIENT OUTCOME/PATHOPHYSIOLOGY

There are two major causes of vaginal bleeding this late in a pregnancy. Placenta previa is a condition in which the placenta implants itself (at the beginning of pregnancy) too close to the cervical opening. As the mother goes into active labor and her cervix begins to dilate, there is a premature separation or tearing of the placenta away from the wall of the uterus. This leads to vaginal bleeding.

Abruptio placenta is the other cause. In this condition the placenta implants itself in the correct position during early pregnancy. However, during the pregnancy it begins to detach itself from the wall of the uterus. This usually happens before active labor begins. The degree of bleeding is directly related to how much of the placenta separates from the uterine wall.

Both placenta previa and abruptio placenta are serious conditions. They may cause shock in the mother but they also cause a decrease in available oxygen and nutrients for the unborn child.

A few hours after the transport you receive a phone call from hospital staff. They wanted to thank you for your timely notification during transport. It allowed them to have the operating room set up for an emergency delivery. The mother was diagnosed with a serious form of abruptio placenta. She was rushed to surgery where she was given 4 units of blood and underwent an emergency c-section. The baby was a little limp at first and did require IV fluids and assistance with breathing. The premature infant is in the neonatal ICU. Both he and his mother are expected to make a full recovery thanks to your excellent assessment and treatment skills.

1. Pregnant patients in their third trimester who experience hypotension when lying supine are likely experiencing:

    a. supine hypotensive syndrome

    b. supine hypertensive syndrome

    c. uterine inversion syndrome

    d. normal reduction of blood pressure in pregnancy

2. The normal pregnancy is _____ weeks.

    a. 24

    b. 34

    c. 36

    d. 40

3. Which of the following conditions occurs early in pregnancy?

    a. uterine rupture

    b. placenta previa

    c. abruptio placenta

    d. ectopic pregnancy

4. Which of the following wouldn't be a treatment for vaginal bleeding in a pregnant patient in her third trimester?

    a. place a sanitary napkin at the vaginal opening

    b. roll the patient to the left side

    c. treat for shock

    d. pack the vagina to stop life-threatening bleeding

5. Which statement in reference to assessing the unborn baby of a mother in shock is true?

    a. The EMT should use a stethoscope to monitor the fetal heart rate.

    b. The fetal heart rate increases proportionately with the mother's heart rate.

    c. Improvement in the mother usually means improvement for the fetus.

    d. The fetal distress is often gauged by increased movement of the fetus.

6. Which statement regarding blood loss is true?

    a. Blood loss can be accurately determined on-scene.

    b. Signs of shock in a patient where blood loss looks minimal indicates significant blood loss.

    c. Blood loss can be easily determined from the patient and bystanders.

    d. An elevated pulse in a patient with a laceration and apparent minimal blood loss should be attributed to stress or excitement.

7. "PNV" in a patient's list of medications would indicate:

   a. pregnancy not viable

   b. prenatal vitamins

   c. penicillin-V

   d. birth control pills

8. It is not necessary to examine the vaginal area of a third-trimester pregnant patient who is bleeding.

   a. true

   b. false

9. Abruptio placenta is:

   a. implantation of the fertilized egg in the placenta

   b. premature separation of the placenta from the uterine wall

   c. premature separation of the placenta from the ovary

   d. one placenta being shared by two or more fetuses

10. Placenta previa is:

   a. implantation of the fertilized egg in the placenta

   b. premature separation of the placenta from the uterine wall

   c. implantation of the placenta too close to the cervical opening

   d. cervical constriction reducing blood flow to the placenta prior to delivery

27

I AM ABOUT TO HAVE THIS BABY

Objectives

At the conclusion of this scenario, the participant will be able to:

1. List the signs of imminent delivery.

2. Describe the assessment of the obstetric patient.

3. Describe the process of delivering a baby.

SCENARIO

The time is 0325 when you are dispatched to a residence for a woman in labor. You are further advised that the patient's contractions are 5 minutes apart. Your response time to the scene is 8 minutes and the closest hospital is 30 miles away.

1. What is the relationship between her contractions and the distance to the hospital?

   Contractions that are occurring 5 minutes apart and a transport time of 5 minutes would more than likely give you time to safely transport and allow delivery to occur in the hospital. In this case, you are looking at a transport time much longer. While en route, you and your partner should prepare for the fact that you may be delivering a baby.

   You arrive at the scene at 0333. A man who introduces himself as the patient's husband escorts you to the living room, where you find a 28-year-old female lying supine on the sofa. As you approach her, she states, "I am about to have this baby." She further states that she is having severe lower back pain, just above her buttocks.

2. Based upon your general impression of the patient, are there any signs of imminent delivery?

There are two significant findings. Though you have not physically examined the patient, the statement "I am about to have this baby" should not be taken lightly. It is a maternal instinct to know when the time has come for delivery. Additionally, her complaint of severe lower back pain signifies that the baby is probably out of the uterus and in the birth canal, where it is putting pressure on the coccyx.

You introduce yourself and your partner to the patient. In an obviously uncomfortable tone of voice, she tells you her name and that this is her second baby. Her 5-year-old son is staying with his grandmother for the weekend. Her husband is coaching her to breathe as you continue your questioning of the patient. Your initial assessment of the patient reveals a patent airway, adequate breathing, and a strong radial pulse that is slightly elevated. Her skin is warm and moist.

3. Are there any other questions that you would ask the patient at this point?

After completion of your initial assessment, your focused exam of the obstetric patient in labor should center around making the decision to transport or deliver on-scene. In addition to the information already provided to you by the patient, you should inquire about the following:

- *How far along is she in her pregnancy.*
- *Whether or not her bag of waters has ruptured and if so, when.*
- *If she has had routine prenatal care.*
- *If there have been any problems with this or her previous pregnancy.*
- *How far apart are her contractions at this point.*

The patient tells you that her due date was yesterday. She went to her obstetrician the day prior and he told her that she was dilated to 3 cm. As you perform a visual exam of the patient, your partner obtains a set of baseline vital signs, which are: B/P 88/60, pulse: 112, and respirations of 30 and shallow.

4. How do you relate the vital-sign findings to the patient's present condition?

It is typical for a woman, especially in the later stages of her pregnancy, to have a lower than usual blood pressure (systolic usually 10–15 mmHg lower) and increased heart rate (usually 10–15 beats/min. faster). These changes are due to an overall increase in the mother's blood volume as well as an increase in maternal cardiac output to meet the oxygen demands of the fetus.

Upon visual exam of the vagina, you note a bulging of the vulva, but do not see any signs of the baby's head. The patient tells you that she feels as though she has to move her bowels. Her husband tells you that her contractions are now approximately 3 minutes apart and are regular, lasting approximately 45 seconds. You consult with your partner and make a determination as to your next step.

5. What significant findings have you discovered thus far in your assessment of this patient?

   At this point, you should have noted the following significant findings:

   - *This patient is at 40 weeks gestation.*
   - *She has the urge to move her bowels.*
   - *Her contractions are occurring in short intervals and are regular.*
   - *You note vaginal bulging.*

6. What decision should you and your partner make with regards to the best approach to this situation?

   The prolonged transport time (30 minutes), her contractions that are now 3 minutes apart and regular, and the vaginal bulging (an imminent precursor to crowning) should secure you and your partner's decision to prepare for an on-scene delivery.

   You place the patient in the supine position on the floor, with her knees bent and thighs spread apart. Your partner opens the OB kit and begins to prepare the patient for delivery. At this point, you can see the baby's head bulging from the vaginal opening. You instruct the mother to breath in through her nose and out through her mouth in between contractions. You also tell her not to push unless she is having a contraction.

7. What are the appropriate body substance isolation precautions that you and your partner should observe with this patient?

   You should already have gloves on. In addition, delivery of a baby will potentially expose you to a number of bodily fluids and substances including blood, amniotic fluid, and maternal/fetal feces, all of which can splatter. The appropriate BSI measures in this case should be gloves, a gown, and full facial protection.

   You note the baby's head visible at the vaginal opening; you apply firm but gentle pressure to its head. After the baby's head delivers, you suction its mouth and nose. The baby's upper shoulders deliver as you guide the head downward, then the lower shoulders deliver as you guide the head upwards. After the shoulders deliver, the rest of the baby follows quickly thereafter.

8. What is the rationale for applying pressure to the baby's head as it delivers?

   By applying firm, <u>but gentle</u> pressure to the baby's head, you will prevent an explosive delivery, which could potentially cause trauma to the mother and to the baby's neck. Remember that the baby has an anterior and a posterior fontanel (soft spots). You want to avoid any and all pressure on these areas.

9. Why not wait until the baby is fully delivered prior to suctioning?

   It is critical to clear as much fetal lung fluid from the child as possible. As the baby travels through the birth canal, its thoracic cavity will be compressed, which will result in the expulsion of fluid from its lungs. By suctioning (mouth first, then the nose) as soon as the head has delivered, you will prevent aspiration of this fluid back into the baby's lungs.

Your partner is applying 100 percent oxygen to the mother. You dry the baby off thoroughly and quickly assess its ABCs, which reveals a healthy-appearing infant with a strong cry and a heart rate of 140. Its hands and feet are blue, but its face and trunk are rapidly "pinking up." You look at the umbilical cord and note that it is not pulsating, after which you clamp and cut it.

10. Why note the cessation of cord pulsation prior to clamping and cutting it?

    Cessation of a pulsating umbilical cord signifies that the vessels supplying the baby with oxygenated blood from the mother are now constricted and no longer patent; therefore, the baby is now oxygenating its own blood and the cord can be safely clamped and cut. In addition, you must also assure that the baby is breathing adequately prior to cutting its "lifeline."

You are now holding a healthy, pink, crying little girl. After completing your assessment of the baby, you wrap it in blankets and hand it to your partner. You note the AP-GAR score at an 8 after 1 minute and 9 after 5 minutes. A police officer has arrived on scene and you ask him to retrieve your stretcher. You and your partner agree that it is time to transport.

While en route, the mother is holding the baby as you monitor her for bleeding as well as delivery of the placenta. You note very little vaginal bleeding and no signs of placental delivery.

11. Why not wait for the placenta to deliver at the scene?

    First of all, you have delivered the most important part, the baby! Second, it can take up to 30 minutes for the placenta to deliver. This can safely be done in the back of the ambulance while en route to the hospital. Time should not be spent at the scene waiting for placental delivery.

12. How would you manage this patient, should you note significant vaginal bleeding?

    There are two ways of managing this situation. First, you can firmly massage the fundus of the uterus. The fundus is the uppermost part of the uterus, which, now that she has delivered, can be palpated just above the umbilicus. Uterine massage will result in vasoconstriction, thereby minimizing any bleeding. You can also allow the baby to breastfeed, which will cause the mother to secrete a chemical in the brain that also results in vasoconstriction. If the bleeding is severe (estimated at more than 500 cc's), you must treat the mother for shock. Remember, you must never pack any dressings into the vagina in an attempt to control bleeding.

Since you are busy with your two patients in the back of the ambulance, you advise your partner to notify the hospital of your ETA. After an uneventful transport, you deliver both mom and baby safely to the emergency department.

PATIENT OUTCOME/PATHOPHYSIOLOGY

After 2 days in the hospital, both mother and baby are discharged from the hospital after an uneventful stay.

For the purposes of this case study, we will discuss only the pathophysiology of the labor process, beginning with the second stage. The EMT can refer to other resources for a review of the entire gestational process.

At the onset of the second stage of labor, the cervix (the inferior opening of the uterus) is fully dilated to 10 cm. Since the EMT cannot determine this without a digital examination (not within the scope of practice of the EMT), the second stage of labor is considered to begin when the baby's head is crowning through the vaginal opening. It is during this stage that the patient will feel the urge to push and/or move her bowels as a result of the baby applying posterior pressure on her rectum.

As the baby travels through the birth canal, its thoracic cavity is compressed, thereby expelling large volumes of amniotic fluid from its lungs. This is why it is important for the EMT to suction the baby's mouth and nose upon delivery of the head. The initial breaths that the baby will take must be free and clear of fetal lung fluid.

As the baby is fully delivered, it is quickly dried, warmed, resuctioned, and assessed, with further management based upon the assessment findings. Birth of the baby ends the second stage of labor and begins the third stage. Once the umbilical cord stops pulsating and the baby is breathing spontaneously and effectively, the cord can safely be clamped and cut.

After initial care and management is provided to the newborn, transport of the mother should begin, with the placenta being allowed to deliver en route to the hospital. The placenta generally takes approximately 30 minutes to deliver. The patient will have a brief return of contractions as the placenta begins to deliver. Delivery of the placenta signals the end of the third stage of labor. The EMT must save the placenta in the plastic bag provided in the OB kit and take it to the hospital where it can be examined for completeness.

Postpartum bleeding is common and expected and is the result of the small blood vessels that hold the placenta to the uterine wall being torn as the placenta detaches. If the blood loss exceeds an estimated 500 cc's, the patient should be evaluated and managed for possible shock.

EVALUATION

1. Which of the following is a sign of imminent delivery?
   a. an overwhelming urge to urinate
   b. contractions that are less than 10 minutes apart
   c. coccygeal pressure and the urge to defecate
   d. irregular contractions that vary in duration

2. During your assessment of a patient with contractions that are 3 minutes apart, lasting 45 seconds, you notice the appearance of the baby's head at the vaginal opening. You should manage this situation appropriately by:
   a. facilitating delivery of the head by gently pulling on it
   b. applying firm pressure to the baby's head until the next contraction begins
   c. inserting two fingers into the vagina in order to establish the baby's airway
   d. applying firm but gentle pressure to the baby's head, avoiding the fontanels

3. Which of the following questions is least helpful in your determination to transport or deliver the baby at the scene?
    a. How far apart are your contractions?
    b. Have you had routine prenatal care?
    c. How far away from the hospital am I?
    d. Do you feel the urge to push?

4. As soon as the baby's head delivers, the EMT should:
    a. suction the nose, then mouth
    b. suction the mouth, then nose
    c. suction the mouth only
    d. suction the nose only

5. During the later stages of pregnancy, which of the following maternal vital sign changes can be expected?
    a. increased blood pressure
    b. decreased heart rate
    c. increased heart rate
    d. no change in blood pressure

6. After delivery of the placenta, you note that the mother is having severe vaginal bleeding, which you estimate to be approximately 700 cc's. She also becomes tachycardic and diaphoretic. In managing this situation, you should:
    a. pack the vagina with sterile dressing as you massage the uterus
    b. elevate the mother's lower extremities 8–12 inches and apply oxygen
    c. place the mother in semisitting position and apply oxygen
    d. apply firm, direct pressure to the area just below the umbilicus

7. In delivering the baby's upper shoulders, the EMT should:
    a. gently pull on the baby's head
    b. guide the baby's head upward
    c. guide the baby's head downward
    d. slightly twist the baby's head to the side

8. You have just delivered a baby, assessed it as being stable, and have clamped and cut the umbilical cord. Your next step should be to:
    a. transport to the hospital
    b. wait for the placenta to deliver
    c. allow the parents to transport the child
    d. call for ALS assistance to start an IV on the mother

9. The third stage of labor begins with:
   a. the onset of contractions
   b. the delivery of the placenta
   c. the birth of the baby
   d. the cessation of umbilical cord pulsation

10. The second stage of labor ends when:
    a. the baby's head is crowning
    b. the cervix is fully dilated
    c. the baby is fully delivered
    d. the placenta has delivered

28

AMPUTATION

Objectives

At the conclusion of this scenario, the participant will be able to:

1. List the assessment steps for a patient with an amputated body part.

2. Describe the management of the patient who has suffered an amputation.

3. Describe the handling techniques of the amputated body part.

SCENARIO

At 1440, your unit is dispatched to a local school woodworking shop, where a student amputated his left hand while working with a table saw. When you arrive at the scene, you are met by the woodworking teacher, who hands you a rolled up paper towel, which he states holds the amputated hand. You hear the patient screaming, "I cut my hand off!"

1. What is your initial priority of management in this situation?

   Even though the amputated part will require special handling in order to maximize the chances of a successful reattachment, life does take priority over limb; therefore, you must gain access to the patient to assess him for severe bleeding and shock.

   The teacher escorts you to the patient, who you find to be a 16-year-old male. You notice that a towel with blood dripping from it is wrapped around his left wrist. The patient's appearance is pale and he is in obvious pain.

2. What have you learned in terms of the general impression of this patient?

   Potential shock. The blood dripping from the towel indicates that this patient is actively bleeding. His pale skin color is an early sign of shock. You must be prepared to initiate shock management for this patient after your initial assessment.

You begin the initial assessment of the patient as your partner applies additional dressings to the bleeding stump. Your assessment findings are as follows:

- Airway open and patent
- Respirations slightly shallow at 26
- Palpable radial pulse in the uninjured extremity with a fast rate
- Obvious bleeding from the covered wound

After tightly wrapping a pressure bandage to the patient's wound, you note that the bleeding is controlled. The patient states that he feels nauseous and is in a tremendous amount of pain. Your partner is applying 100 percent oxygen via nonrebreather to the patient.

3. Had the pressure bandage not controlled the bleeding, what other techniques would you have employed?

    Recall the steps of controlling bleeding in their order of preference:

    - *Direct pressure*
    - *Elevation*
    - *Pressure bandage*
    - *Pressure-point control*
    - *Tourniquet*

    If the pressure bandage had been unsuccessful, the appropriate next step in management would have been applying pressure to a proximal pressure point. In this case, the brachial artery would have been the site of choice as it is closest to the wound.

The patient tells you that he was cutting a piece of wood with the table saw, when the wood jammed in the blade. When he attempted to free the piece of wood, it dislodged and cut his hand off. He denies any other injury. Your partner takes a set of baseline vital signs, which are: BP 140/80, pulse 124/strong, respirations 26 and slightly shallow.

4. What additional injury might this patient have received based upon the mechanism of injury?

    Due to the twisting motion of the table saw, you should be suspicious of possible fracture or dislocation to the elbow as well as the shoulder. With the trauma that this patient has experienced, he may not feel the pain of other injuries.

5. What patient priority category should this patient be placed in?

    Due to the fact that there is a narrow window (approximately 4 hours) for successfully reimplanting the patient's hand as well as the fact that he is showing potential early signs of shock (i.e., pallor), this patient should be treated as a priority patient and transport should occur without delay.

You perform a quick rapid assessment of the patient, which reveals no further injury or abnormalities aside from a few abrasions to his left forearm. Meanwhile, your partner retrieves the amputated hand from the shop teacher.

6. What should your management of the amputated hand consist of?

The amputated hand should be wrapped in a sterile dressing, which is placed into a plastic bag, then the bag should be placed on ice. Direct contact of the amputated part with the ice should be avoided, as this will cause damage to the tissue and cells of the hand, thereby minimizing the chance of a successful reimplantation. Additionally, the amputated part should not be submerged in saline or other solutions. If the amputation is incomplete, it should be bandaged and splinted in the position found. You should never complete a partial amputation. The goal is to keep the amputated part viable without causing further damage.

After providing the appropriate care for the amputated hand, you place the patient on the stretcher and begin transport of the patient to a hospital that is 12 miles away. The amputated hand is transported with the patient.

7. Would your management of the patient have changed had you not been able to locate the amputated part?

Although every attempt should be made to locate and properly handle the amputated part, expedient patient care should not suffer because of it. Your treatment of the patient for potential shock and prompt transport should happen whether the amputated part is retrieved or not.

En route to the hospital, you obtain a SAMPLE history from the patient. The only pertinent finding is that he states he is allergic to tetanus toxoid.

8. What is the correlation between his allergy to a tetanus shot and his injury?

Patients that sustain injuries such as this will in all likelihood receive a tetanus booster in the emergency department as prophylaxis. Even though this finding will not change your management of the patient, it is pertinent information to pass on to the emergency department staff.

While transporting the patient, you are consistently monitoring him. You call a report in to the destination facility and apprise them of the situation and your estimated time of arrival.

9. What should you be monitoring the patient for while en route to the hospital?

You should be monitoring this patient for further signs of progressing shock such as increasing anxiety and restlessness, thirst, and the development hypotension. In addition, you must constantly monitor the pressure bandage to ensure that blood is not soaking through the dressing. Since you are handling this as a critical situation, the ongoing assessment should be repeated every 5 minutes. The nature of the injury will certainly require compassionate care, too.

PATIENT OUTCOME/PATHOPHYSIOLOGY

After a lengthy surgery to attempt to reattach the patient's hand, the surgeon's best attempts were unsuccessful. He was kept in the hospital for 7 days of antibiotic therapy and then discharged home.

An amputation occurs when a part of the body (usually an extremity or part thereof) is traumatically detached from the body. The most common mechanisms of injury for an amputation are crushing injuries such as those sustained in a motor vehicle crash and industrial accidents, such as the one described in this case study. The immediate risk to the patient from an amputation is severe external hemorrhage and shock; however, the bleeding is not always as severe as one would expect. This is because of the sensitivity of the vasculature to ambient air. For example, if a portion of an extremity is amputated, the blood vessels will constrict and draw back into the remaining stump of the extremity, thereby limiting the amount of external bleeding. Even though the bleeding can still be severe in cases where a large major artery is disrupted and may require the application of a tourniquet, usually the bleeding can be controlled with the application of a tightly wrapped pressure dressing. A secondary risk to the patient is infection. This risk can be minimized in the field if the EMT follows proper aseptic technique. Generally speaking, there is a window of 4–6 hours in which the extremity can be reimplanted; therefore, it is critical that the EMT handle the amputated part with care, which includes wrapping it in a sterile dressing, placing it in a plastic bag, and placing the bag on ice. Do not allow the extremity to freeze.

EVALUATION

1. A construction worker has amputated his left arm just below the elbow when a steel girder fell on it. As you approach the patient, you note that he is seriously bleeding from the area of detachment. As you assess and manage the patient's airway, your partner should:

   a. call for ALS assistance
   b. control the bleeding
   c. keep the patient warm
   d. elevate the patient's legs

2. The initial means of controlling bleeding from an amputated extremity is to:
   a. apply a tourniquet
   b. apply pressure point control
   c. firmly apply direct pressure
   d. apply a pressure bandage

3. You are managing a patient with an amputated lower extremity. The location of the amputated leg is unknown. The patient begins to exhibit signs and symptoms of shock. You should:

   a. find the amputated leg before you transport the patient to the hospital
   b. have a police officer locate the leg, pack it on ice, and bring it to the hospital
   c. complete only the necessary management at the scene and immediately transport
   d. request an ALS assistance to start an IV in order to give you time to locate the leg

4. Appropriate care for an amputated extremity includes:

   a. packing the extremity in ice and transporting with the patient

   b. placing the extremity on top of dry ice and transporting it with the patient

   c. keeping the extremity warm with chemical heat packs and transporting it with the patient

   d. wrapping the extremity in sterile dressing, placing it in a plastic bag, and placing the bag on ice

5. You are transporting a patient with an amputated right arm. Management for this patient includes all of the following EXCEPT:

   a. telling the patient that they will be able to reattach his arm

   b. continually assessing the patient for signs/symptoms of shock

   c. transporting the patient to the closest appropriate facility

   d. reassuring the patient while en route to the hospital

6. A patient has partially amputated his left index finger in an incident with a meat grinder. Appropriate management for this patient includes:

   a. bandage and splint the finger as is

   b. complete the amputation with your scissors

   c. soak his entire hand in sterile saline

   d. pack his entire hand in ice and transport

7. Which of the following most accurately describes the reaction of the blood vessels as an extremity is amputated?

   a. the blood vessels dilate and increase the severity of the bleeding

   b. the blood vessels constrict and draw back into the stump

   c. the blood vessels dilate and draw back into the stump

   d. there is no reaction of the vasculature to an amputation

8. The appropriate artery to apply pressure to, should your initial efforts to control the bleeding from an amputated hand fail, is the:

   a. radial

   b. popliteal

   c. femoral

   d. brachial

9. Your primary concern when managing a patient with an amputated extremity should be to:

   a. locate the amputated part

   b. treat the patient for shock

   c. protect the patient from infection secondary to the injury

   d. determine whether the amputation is full or incomplete

10. While transporting a patient with an amputated leg who is in shock, he should be reassessed:

a. every 5 minutes

b. every 10 minutes

c. every 15 minutes

d. only if his condition worsens

29

I Cut My Hand

Objectives

At the conclusion of this scenario, the participant will be able to:

1. Describe the assessment for a patient with a soft tissue injury.

2. Define the steps of management for a soft tissue injury.

3. Recognize the importance of aseptic technique while managing a soft tissue injury.

SCENARIO

At 1930, your unit is dispatched to a local supermarket where a man has evidently cut his hand while cutting up beef. The dispatcher advises you that the patient is conscious and alert.

1. What types of injuries might this patient have sustained, given the dispatch information?

   Given the dispatch information, this patient could have simply cut his hand with a butcher knife or sustained a mutilating hand injury from a meat grinder. Either way, you should prepare for the worst type of injury. Don't forget your body substance isolation precautions.

   You arrive at the scene at 1936 with your PPE donned. You enter the rear of the supermarket where you find the patient, a 36-year-old male, whose hand is wrapped in a towel. You do not see any evidence of blood on the towel.

   Your initial assessment reveals a conscious and alert patient with adequate breathing and a palpable radial pulse, which seems fast. His skin is pink, warm, and dry. There are no other signs of obvious injury or bleeding.

2. With a hand injury significant enough to warrant the summoning of EMS, wouldn't you expect to see signs of a more severe injury (e.g., blood-soaked towel)?

First of all, you haven't exposed the wound in order to determine its severity. Furthermore, for all you know, a bystander may have given the patient another towel after the previous one became blood-soaked. Remember, things are not always as they appear. Clearly a more detailed assessment is needed.

3. What most likely accounts for the patient's fast radial pulse?

In this case, pain is the most likely cause of his tachycardia. Remember, early signs of shock include restlessness, diaphoresis, and tachycardia. Physiologically, if this patient was going into shock, you would likely see signs other than tachycardia alone, none of which the patient is displaying.

Recognizing that a focused exam is the most appropriate approach to the patient, you expose the wound as your partner is obtaining a set of baseline vital signs on the opposite extremity. Upon exposing the injury site, you note a laceration through the palm of the hand, which is approximately 1 1/2 inches in length and approximately 1/2 inch in depth. Minimal amounts of dark red blood begin flowing from the wound. He is able to easily move his fingers and his capillary refill time is approximately 1 second.

The patient tells you that he was "quartering" a side of beef when the knife slipped and cut his hand. A coworker further tells you that he immediately wrapped the patient's hand with a towel and moved him outside to the loading dock. Your partner reports that the patient's blood pressure is 130/90, pulse is 112, and respirations are 14 and eupneic.

4. What questions would be appropriate to ask this patient, based on the mechanism in which he sustained the injury?

In addition to the routine SAMPLE history obtained on all patients, this patient should be questioned as to when he received his last tetanus shot. Due to the obviously contaminated knife, not only is he at risk of infection, but also tetanus, which can be life threatening.

5. What does your partner mean when he says that the patient's respirations are "eupneic"?

The term "eupnea" refers to respirations that are normal in rate, regularity, and quality. In other words, the patient is breathing adequately.

You dress and bandage the patient's hand with sterile 4 × 4 gauze pads and roller gauze, after which you check the capillary refill in the injured hand and ask the patient to wiggle his fingers. Capillary refill time is approximately 1 second and he is able to move his fingers.

6. Why not palpate the radial pulse after you have dressed and bandaged the patient's hand? Isn't it a distal pulse?

In relationship to the injury, the radial pulse is a proximal, not distal. You must always assess distal sensory, motor, and circulation in an injured extremity before and after dressing and bandaging.

7. What does the rapid capillary refill and the ability of the patient to move his fingers tell you?

These findings tell you two things. First, there is no neurologic compromise distal to the injury and second, he is getting adequate blood flow distal to the injury. If the capillary re-fill time was delayed and/or the patient could not move his fingers, the wound may have caused nerve and vascular damage or you may have inadvertently applied the dressing too tight.

After completing your management of the patient's injured hand and obtaining the information for your patient care form, he requests that you take him to a nearby hospital. A coworker offers to take the patient in his car.

8. What is your most appropriate response to the patient's request and the coworker's willingness to take the patient in his car?

Even though the patient's injury is clearly not life threatening, EMS should transport all patients to the hospital who request it, no matter how minor the injury might appear. Convincing the patient to go to the hospital in his coworker's car could come back to haunt you as abandonment.

As you are walking the patient to the ambulance, he changes his mind and tells you that he can't afford the ambulance bill and would rather go with his friend. You advise the patient that you would gladly transport him, yet he still refuses. After informing the patient of the potential risks of refusal, you obtain a signed refusal and then return your unit to service.

PATIENT OUTCOME/PATHOPHYSIOLOGY

After signing your refusal form, the patient's coworker took him to a nearby emergency department, where his wound was cleaned and sutured. There was no underlying major vascular or neurological damage. The patient was discharged home.

Soft tissue injuries can range from simple abrasions to massive open wounds with severe bleeding and shock. Lacerations are among the most common soft tissue injuries encountered by the EMT. A laceration is caused by a sharp object that produces a jagged injury with varying degrees of length and depth. The severity of the injury is dependent upon the area of the body injured as well as the depth of the laceration. Potential complications from this type of injury include severe bleeding and potential shock, underlying vascular, nerve, and tendon damage, as well as infection. EMS care will depend upon the severity of injury. Bleeding should be controlled initially with direct pressure. If this is not effective, elevation, pressure dressing, pressure-point control, and, as a last resort, a tourniquet should be applied. Typical care in the emergency department includes thorough cleaning of the wound, suturing, a tetanus booster, and occasionally, prophylactic antibiotics.

EVALUATION

1. Which of the following best describes the characteristics of a laceration?
   a. an injury with smooth edges
   b. an injury with jagged edges
   c. an injury that produces a flap of tissue
   d. an injury in which the skin is scraped from the epidermis

2. The most significant initial complication of a severe laceration is:
   a. massive infection
   b. underlying nerve damage
   c. bleeding and shock
   d. permanent disfigurement

3. Your first consideration when caring for a patient with a large laceration to the forehead is:
   a. direct pressure to the injury
   b. a tightly wrapped pressure bandage
   c. 100 percent oxygen with a nonrebreather mask
   d. body substance isolation precautions

4. Dark red blood that is freely flowing from a hand laceration is indicative of:
   a. arterial bleeding
   b. venous bleeding
   c. capillary bleeding
   d. the most serious type of bleeding

5. A 20-year-old male has sustained a 2-inch laceration, with minimal bleeding, to the medial aspect of his left forearm. He is conscious and alert with palpable radial pulses at a rate of 112 and strong. His skin is pink, warm, and dry. What is the most likely cause of the tachycardia in this particular patient?
   a. pain and/or anxiety
   b. compensated shock
   c. decompensated shock
   d. severe internal bleeding

6. The preferred initial means to control external bleeding from a laceration to the mid-forearm is with the use of:
   a. direct pressure
   b. elevation of the arm
   c. a pressure bandage
   d. pressure to the brachial artery

7. You have bandaged a laceration to a patient's left hand. Prior to the bandaging, distal circulation as well as sensory and motor function was intact. Now the patient complains of tingling to the fingers and you note that his hand is somewhat cool. What has probably happened?

   a. vascular and nerve damage due to the injury
   b. the bandage was applied too loosely
   c. the bandage was applied too tightly
   d. an increase in blood flow distal to the injury

8. To manage the situation described in question 7, the EMT should:

   a. elevate the extremity and transport
   b. tighten the bandage to the wound
   c. loosen the bandage to the wound
   d. keep the extremity lower than the heart

9. After dressing and bandaging a laceration to the upper leg of a young male patient, you notice that blood is rapidly soaking through the bandage. You should:

   a. apply a tourniquet
   b. apply more dressings
   c. apply pressure to the popliteal artery
   d. remove the dressing to evaluate the wound

10. The most distal pulse to check in a patient with a laceration to the antecubital fossa (the anterior bend of the elbow) is the:

    a. brachial pulse
    b. femoral pulse
    c. radial pulse
    d. dorsalis pedis pulse

30

I'VE BURNED MYSELF

Objectives

At the conclusion of this scenario, the participant will be able to:

1. List the classification of burns.

2. Describe the components of the "Rules of 9."

3. Discuss treatment objectives for burn victims.

SCENARIO

Your ambulance has been dispatched to a private residence for a man who has been burned. The caller reported that her husband suffered burns while attempting to light a barbecue grill. He could be heard screaming in the background. The call is less than two blocks from the station. You should arrive on scene in less than 2 minutes.

1. What are your thoughts concerning this dispatch information? Should other agencies be notified?

You are aware that the patient is an adult male who has suffered a thermal injury. However, we are not yet aware as to which part of his body was burned and to what extent he is burned. He is conscious at the time of the call. You would be prudent to request fire department response. This type of call is very vague in nature. We do not know whether or not the fire may have spread to other structures. It is always easier to cancel nonnecessary units than to need them and have them delayed or not available.

2. What is your first priority upon arrival at the scene?

Without a doubt, safety. You must ensure your safety and that of your partner to effectively help the patient. If you or your partner become injured then you have only compounded the problem. You must ensure that the source of thermal injury has not spread and that the fire has been extinguished.

You arrive on scene. Before exiting the ambulance you and your partner put on your BSI equipment, which includes your gloves and eye protection at a minimum. You grab your first-in bag and your burn kit before you approach the home. You can hear someone screaming from the backyard. You and your partner cautiously move in that direction. As you round the corner of the house you see a man standing on the patio. His right arm appears blackened and is still smoldering.

3. What is your next immediate priority?

Stop the burning process. This patient has suffered a thermal injury to his right arm and it continues to burn. This is evidenced by the smoldering appearance. You should extinguish the burning process caused by flames by wetting the area with tap water, sterile water, or normal saline. If not available then you should smother the area that continues to burn. Clothing should be removed. Burns that are caused by items such as grease, wax, tar, or paraffins are treated somewhat differently. These items should not be removed. Simply stop the burning process by cooling with water.

You instruct your partner to get the garden hose and turn on the water. As your partner carries out your instructions you approach the patient. You ask him where he is hurt. He tells you that he was pouring some lighter fluid on the barbecue grill when it suddenly caught his shirt and arm on fire. He thinks that this is the only area he is burned. He says that the shirt is continuing to burn. You and your partner begin to run water on the arm. You are able to determine that the burning process has stopped since there is no further smoldering evident. You also remove his shirt to ensure that it doesn't reignite. The patient is in serious pain. You instruct your partner to open up the burn dressings.

4. What is the next step in your care?

You need to perform your assessment. We are unable to tell as of yet whether or not there are other areas of injury that might take priority over the arm. This is referred to as "distracting injuries." We must remember to assess all patients in an organized, step-by-step fashion to avoid missing other injuries.

You begin your focused history and physical exam. You have already determined that the patient is awake and alert. His airway is open and he is breathing adequately. He does have radial pulses noted on both arms. You sit the patient down on a patio chair so that you can calm him down. You perform your head-to-toe assessment. You note that both of the patient's eyebrows have singed hair. You see that the front of his hairline is also singed.

5. What should you assess for next?

You should assess the airway for signs and symptoms of inhalation injury. Since you have witnessed singed facial hair you are aware that his face was also exposed to potential thermal injury. This means that he could have inhaled "super-heated" air or gasses into his lungs. You must assess him for complications that could result from this type of injury. Be cognizant of soft tissue charring and swelling. Signs such as sooty sputum production or a stridorous airway are potentially dangerous warning signs.

You assess the victim's airway. You don't see singed nasal hairs or sooty material on his tongue. No soft tissue swelling is evident. His respirations are clear and nonlabored. You assess the neck and see no evidence of burns or trauma. You have already bared his chest when you took off his shirt. There are no burns noted to the thorax. Bilateral breath sounds are clear to auscultation. The abdomen is soft with no evidence of burns. The patient is wearing blue jeans and no injury was sustained to the lower extremities. The back is also clear. The left arm appears uninjured. However, the right arm has sustained substantial thermal injury. It appears that the patient has circumferential burns that involve everything from the fingers up to an area about 1 inch from the shoulder. Much of the area is charred black in color with some of the upper arm bright red with blistering noted.

6. How do we classify burns?

Burns are generally classified by the source of injury and by the depth of injury. For example, thermal injuries generally result from fire or super-heated gasses such as steam. Burns may also occur secondary to an electrical injury or chemical exposure. If chemicals are involved, try to ascertain what type of chemical it was. Treatment may be different depending upon which chemicals are involved. As far as the depth of injury, we used to utilize old terms like first-, second-, or third-degree burns. We have since changed our taxonomy to include the following terms: superficial, partial thickness, or full thickness burns. Superficial means that only the outer layer of skin (epidermis) is involved. This is evident by redness only. Partial-thickness burns completely burn through the epidermis and actually injure the dermis as well. Severe pain is generally reported. These burns are evidenced by severe redness along with blister formation. Full-thickness burns burn completely through the epidermis and dermal layers and may involve fat, muscle, or bone layers. Most patients are unable to feel pain directly at the full-thickness burn site; however, the surrounding tissues, which have lesser degree of burns, are generally very painful. The full-thickness burns may appear charred black, dark brown, or patchy white and yellow in color. Also be aware that children and geriatrics that suffer burns have a higher risk of complications.

7. What percentage of the body has been burned?

Burns are also described by the percent of total body surface area (TBSA) that is involved. Utilizing this method, the palm of the patient is equivalent to about 1 percent. Another method, which has been precalculated, is called the "Rules of 9." The percent of each area is different for adults, children, and infants because of disproportionate sizes during different stages of development. The Rules of 9 for adults are as follows:

RULES OF NINE		
	Front	Back
Head	4½%	4½%
Chest	9%	9%
Abdomen	9%	9%
Genitalia	1%	
Right Leg	9%	9%
Left Leg	9%	9%
Right Arm	4½%	4½%
Left Arm	4½%	4½%

8. How would you describe these burns?

   You have identified that a majority of the right arm is involved and the burn is circumferential. By utilizing the Rules of 9 you estimate that approximately 9 percent of the TBSA is involved. This should also be classified as a thermal burn secondary to flame. The depth of burn should be described as mostly full-thickness with some areas of partial-thickness burns.

   You begin to dress the wound with burn dressings after you delicately weave sterile 4 × 4 gauze between the webs of his fingers. The patient's wife asks if you want some "butter" to place on the burns to help reduce the pain.

9. What type of dressing will be applied? Will you utilize the butter offered by the spouse?

   Since you have stopped the burning process you should now place a dry, sterile burn dressing over the injured extremity. (Some systems allow wet dressings if less than 10 percent BSA is involved.) You would never use butter or any other item to place directly on a burn. The practice of using butter for burns is an old one and still engrained in many cultures. It is true that it does reduce pain, but at the cost of keeping thermal energy trapped in the wound. This promotes further burning and injury deeper in the wound. Other home remedies include shaving cream and cooking oil. These too should be avoided.

   After completing your dressing application you assist the patient to the stretcher. Your partner applies oxygen to the patient at 15 Lpm with a nonrebreather mask. You begin to move the patient to the ambulance as you gather your SAMPLE history. You find that the patient has no allergies and takes no medications. He also has no past medical history. He was just about to begin cooking supper so he hasn't eaten in several hours. Once in the ambulance you assess his vital signs, which are as follows: B/P 148/90, HR 124, RR 22, and an SpO_2 of 99 percent on oxygen.

   You immediately begin transport to the closest hospital when you are told to reroute to the trauma center. You are aware that they have done this because the trauma center also houses a burn unit, which specializes in severe burns. You transport the patient the extra 5 minutes to the trauma center where a team is awaiting your arrival. You deliver your patient and report and return to service.

PATIENT OUTCOME/PATHOPHYSIOLOGY

The patient was initially managed in the emergency department of the trauma center with IV fluid resuscitation and pain medication before being transferred upstairs to the burn unit. There he underwent debridement of the arm. It was calculated that 8 percent of his TBSA was burned. Full-thickness burns of 6½ percent and 1½ percent partial-thickness burns were noted. He was hospitalized for over a month, during which time he underwent numerous debridements and skin-grafting procedures. He did lose four of his five fingers despite aggressive treatment. He will be discharged next week but will undergo months of rehabilitation and physical therapy.

EVALUATION

1. Burns that are characterized by reddened skin only are most likely:
   a. superficial burns
   b. partial-thickness burns
   c. full-thickness burns
   d. eschar burns

2. Burns that are characterized by black charred skin with no sense of feeling are known as:
   a. superficial burns
   b. partial-thickness burns
   c. full-thickness burns
   d. eschar burns

3. Burns that are characterized by bright red skin with blisters are known as:
   a. superficial burns
   b. partial-thickness burns
   c. full-thickness burns
   d. eschar burns

4. Burns that involve the front of both legs would make up what percent of TBSA, utilizing the Rules of 9 assessment?
   a. 4½ percent
   b. 9 percent
   c. 18 percent
   d. 27 percent

5. Burns that involve all of the anterior chest and abdomen along with the upper back would make up what percent of TBSA, utilizing the Rules of 9 assessment?

   a. 9 percent
   b. 18 percent
   c. 27 percent
   d. 36 percent

6. Which of these would cause suspicion of an inhalation injury?

   a. singed nasal hairs
   b. sooty material on tongue and throat
   c. stridorous breathing sounds
   d. all of the above

7. What is your first priority at the scene of a thermal injury?

   a. put out the fire
   b. your own scene safety
   c. calculate the Rules of 9
   d. determine the agent that caused the burn

8. Burn victims are best cared for by a burn center.

   a. true
   b. false

9. Which of the following items are acceptable to put on burns to reduce the severity of pain?

   a. shaving cream
   b. cooking oil
   c. butter
   d. none of the above

10. Which of the following items should be removed if they are on an extremity that has been burned?

    a. clothing
    b. watches
    c. rings
    d. all of the above

31

I'VE CUT MY ARM WITH A SAW

Objectives

At the conclusion of this scenario, the participant will be able to:

1. Discuss the assessment of severe soft tissue injuries.

2. List treatment options available to reduce severe bleeding.

3. Identify appropriate use of tourniquet application.

SCENARIO

Your ambulance has been dispatched to a residence where a man called "911" from his wood shop, stating that he had cut his arm with a circular saw. You have a 4-minute ETA to the scene.

1. What are your thoughts regarding the dispatch information?

   Dispatch stated that the caller reported his own injury. That means that at the time of call he was alert and able to summon his own help. The dispatcher also reported that a circular saw was the item inflicting injury. Circular saws are hand-held electrical saws that have a circular rotating blade. They turn very rapidly and have a menacing saw-tooth pattern. They are capable of causing severe injury to soft tissue, muscles, tendons, ligaments, and even bone. They are commonly the cause of digit amputations.

2. What should you do en route to prepare for this call?

   You should first prepare by applying your personal protective equipment. You should wear gloves and eye protection at a minimum. The risk for arterial injury is high and you need to protect yourself from unnecessary exposure to blood and body fluids. You should also consider which bags you will be carrying to the patient. If your service has a separate bag for trauma then you should definitely include that with your other equipment.

You arrive on scene in front of the residence. You are very observant for scene safety considerations. You see that there is a small work shed behind the home. You see someone sitting on a chair holding a towel that appears to be blood soaked. He is writhing in pain.

3. What are your thoughts concerning this limited scene observation?

Simply put: blood loss. You see that the victim is sitting upright and writhing in pain. That means that he remains conscious and possibly alert. The blood-soaked towel is your greatest concern. You should be prepared to handle a patient who may be in hemorrhagic shock.

You cautiously enter the work shed. There you see a circular saw that is lying on the floor. It is silent and not operating at present. You are able to see copious amounts of blood on the wall, ceiling, floor, and pooling underneath the patient. You approach the patient and begin your patient assessment. After securing consent you immediately perform your initial assessment. You have already identified that the patient is conscious and alert. His airway is open and he is breathing rapidly. He has a weak and rapid radial pulse on the un-affected arm. He is holding a towel tightly around his left forearm. He continues to bleed through the towel.

4. What is your next priority?

Stop the bleeding. Continued blood loss will only worsen or increase the likelihood of shock. It is apparent that the towel has not been successful in stopping the bleeding. You may have to employ several maneuvers to limit bleeding. Since the towel is not helping, you must observe the injury site and apply a new dressing. Remember that a dressing is something that is in direct contact with the wound. A bandage is something that holds the dressing in place. After examining the wound you should apply direct pressure, with your dressing, to the bleeding injury. Other techniques that may help slow the bleeding include raising the ex-tremity above the level of the heart, application of cold compresses, pressure dressing appli-cation, pressure points of the vascular system, and finally tourniquet application.

The patient reports that this is an isolated injury. He is actively bleeding so you de-cide to examine the injury by removing the towel from his forearm. You open a multi-trauma dressing so that you will be prepared. You see a large, gaping laceration with significant tissue damage. The laceration is approximately 7 inches long and at least 2 inches wide. You are able to see bone and many other structures. Immediately there is a stream of pulsatile blood, which is released from the wound. The first wave travels through the air and strikes your partner in the face. You immediately apply a trauma dressing as you begin to apply direct pressure to the site. You also elevate the extremity above the level of the patient's heart. Your partner tells you that some of the blood went above his eyewear and then came down, striking him in the eye.

5. What should you instruct your partner to do?

If there is running water immediately available then you should have him immediately rinse his eye with tap water. Exposure to blood may lead to a transmission of diseases such as hep-atitis and HIV. Hepatitis is the most commonly acquired blood-borne pathogen that health-

care workers come into contact with. It can cause life-long complications. Instruct your partner to wash his eyes immediately if possible.

Your partner immediately goes to the sink and flushes his eyes with water. You continue to assess the effectiveness of your attempt to stop the bleeding.

6. How would you assess for the continuation of bleeding? Would you remove the dressing to examine the wound?

You would assess for bleeding by visualizing your dressing. Does the blood continue to leak through your dressing? Is your trauma dressing saturated? You will not remove your trauma dressing. If you apply a dressing or if a patient has a dressing applied before you arrive and they continue to bleed through then it is acceptable to remove the dressing once to see what is bleeding and reapply another dressing. However, once you have examined the wound and have applied a dressing you will not remove it again. Instead you will continue to reinforce your primary dressing with subsequent dressing and escalate in your interventions to stop the bleeding.

You note that the dressing is completely saturated and blood is leaking through and around it as well. You ask your partner to open more dressings and you reinforce the primary dressing with subsequent dressings. You note that this is a serious laceration and that may require constant care.

7. What have you identified about this situation?

This situation is a true load-and-go emergency. Bleeding that is severe or that cannot be controlled requires immediate transport. You should begin to make efforts to begin transport and perform all other functions en route to the hospital.

You direct your partner to prepare the stretcher and prepare for oxygen administration. You begin to apply roller gauze to the wound in an effort to apply a pressure dressing since your manual pressure was not sufficient. You quickly assist the patient to the stretcher as your partner places him on oxygen at 15 Lpm with a nonrebreather mask. You immediately move him to the ambulance, where you secure him for transport. You note that in that short distance your pressure dressing is again saturated with blood. He continues to bleed.

8. What is your next intervention?

You need to escalate your attempts to stop the bleeding. You have already applied a dressing, applied direct pressure, and attempted to place a pressure dressing. None of these options have been successful. You need to apply pressure to the artery that feeds blood to this area of the body. In this case, since the laceration is located on the forearm, you know that the brachial artery via the upper arm supplies the radial and ulnar arteries. You know that the brachial artery traverses the upper arm, running along the medial aspect between the biceps and triceps. You can apply pressure by manually compressing it between your fingers and the humerus.

You request that your partner go en route to the trauma center, which is 15-minutes away. You also ask that he request another unit or a supervisor to junction with you en route. He immediately begins the emergency transport. You begin to apply pressure to the brachial artery. You continue to apply manual direct pressure over your pressure dressing and elevate the extremity as well. Since you are forced to stay in this position until further help arrives you begin your SAMPLE history. You are able to find out that the patient is 60 years old. He was cutting a wooden plank when the saw hit a knot in the wood causing it to bounce up, striking him in the left arm. He has no allergies to medication. The only medications that he takes are Nifedipine and Coumadin. His past medical history includes an AMI about 3 years ago for which he takes these medications. His last meal was about 2 hours ago and he did not lose consciousness with the event. Your partner reports that he can see the supervisor up ahead and that he is pulling over. You are still about 10 minutes away from the trauma center.

9. Why is it important to gather a SAMPLE history from trauma patients?

This is a prime example. The information gathered in this simple exchange was invaluable. The key in this case is the medications that the patient takes.

Nifedipine (aka Procardia) is a calcium-channel blocker. It is utilized to keep patients with heart conditions from becoming hypertensive and to reduce the stress and workload of the heart.

Coumadin (aka Warfarin) is a blood-thinning agent. Patients who suffer acute heart attacks or strokes may benefit from keeping their blood thinned. It reduces the risk of recurrent heart attacks.

As you can see, the medication that is designed to save the lives of patients is now working against this patient. Coumadin is a potent blood thinner. This patient continues to bleed because his blood is so thin that it is having difficulty clotting. This is a true emergency.

Your supervisor steps up in the back of the ambulance and asks what you would like him to do. You instruct him to perform a quick head-to-toe assessment, assess vital signs and give notification to the trauma center. The head-to-toe exam was unremarkable except for the injury noted. His vital signs are: B/P 90/50, HR 100, RR 22, and an SpO$_2$ of 99 percent on oxygen. You note that despite the pressure being applied to the brachial artery, the patient continues to bleed through the dressing.

10. What is your next intervention for the continued bleeding?

This is the most severe form of bleeding. You will need to employ the most desperate field maneuver to stop the bleeding: tourniquet application. You decide to utilize a blood pressure cuff as the tourniquet. You place a roll of gauze over the brachial artery. You then apply the B/P cuff over the gauze. You then inflate the B/P cuff to stop artery blood flow. Since you know that the B/P was 90mmHg systolic, most experts suggest that you should inflate your B/P cuff to approximately 30–40mmHg above this number. You need to exactly mark what time tourniquets are applied. It should be prominently displayed somewhere on the patient's body. Some texts advocate writing the time of tourniquet application on the patient's forehead.

You apply the tourniquet to the brachial area to stop blood flow to the distal extremity. You arrive at the trauma center within 5 minutes. You give a detailed report to the trauma team. You also direct your partner to begin filling out an "Exposure Report Form" so that he may be tested and treated accordingly for his exposure to blood and body fluids.

You and your supervisor clean the ambulance as you discuss the call. He congratulates you on a job well done.

PATIENT OUTCOME/PATHOPHYSIOLOGY

The patient was assessed by the trauma team. His rapid laboratory assessment revealed that his hemoglobin was 7.5 and his hematocrit was 22. This indicates a severe amount of blood loss. He was treated with doses of vitamin K to counteract the effects of the Coumadin. He was also transfused with 4 units of blood. He was taken to the operating room where it was determined that he lacerated both his radial and ulnar arteries. He underwent extensive surgery to repair his vasculature. He also underwent repair of numerous tendons and ligaments. He will remain in the hospital for several days and will need months of physical therapy to improve the function of his injured arm.

EVALUATION

1. Why do we wear gloves during patient contacts?
    a. to reduce the transmission of our germs to the patient
    b. to reduce the likelihood of exposure to blood and body fluids
    c. to prevent the transmission of hepatitis
    d. to prevent the transmission of HIV

2. What is the most commonly acquired blood-borne pathogen that healthcare workers come into contact with?
    a. herpes
    b. HIV
    c. hepatitis
    d. e. coli

3. What is the device called that is placed directly in contact with an open wound?
    a. band-aid
    b. gauze
    c. bandage
    d. dressing

4. What is the device called that holds the answer to question 3 in place?
    a. band-aid
    b. gauze
    c. bandage
    d. dressing

5. What is the first step in your attempt to stop bleeding?
    a. direct pressure
    b. elevation

c. pressure point

d. tourniquet application

6. What is the last step you may utilize in the field to stop bleeding?

    a. direct pressure

    b. elevation

    c. pressure point

    d. tourniquet application

7. Which of the following medications would interfere with your ability to control bleeding?

    a. Nifedipine

    b. Lanoxin

    c. Coumadin

    d. Procardia

8. How does elevation help to control hemorrhage?

    a. by reducing the force or pressure of blood delivery

    b. it increases the delivery of clotting factors to the site

    c. it stops blood delivery when elevated above the heart

    d. none of the above

9. Which of the following is an indication of arterial laceration?

    a. bright red bleeding

    b. spurting blood

    c. diminished or absent pulse distal to said artery

    d. all of the above

10. Uncontrollable hemorrhage is a load-and-go situation.

    a. true

    b. false

32

MY ARM IS BROKEN

Objectives

At the conclusion of this scenario, the participant will be able to:

1. Describe the assessment of the patient with a musculoskeletal injury.

2. List the signs and symptoms of a musculoskeletal injury.

3. Define the techniques of management for musculoskeletal injuries.

SCENARIO

You are standing by at a local high school volleyball game when you witness an 18-year-old female attempt to return a volley. She falls back, landing on her right arm and hyperflexing her hand. You hear a loud "pop" as she lands. She immediately screams in pain.

1. What are the advantages of your unit being present as the injury occurred?

There are several advantages to your ambulance being present at the time of the injury. First, you will be able to provide care within a matter of seconds. Second, you witnessed the mechanism of injury firsthand. In most cases, EMTs must rely on bystanders or their own formulation of the scene in order to determine how the injury occurred.

As the patient is writhing in pain on the floor, you proceed to her as your partner retrieves the trauma kit. When you arrive at the patient's side, she is holding her right arm up against her chest. She tells you "My arm is broken!" After some reluctance, she allows you to visually inspect her injured arm. You immediately note gross deformity to the distal aspect of her forearm, which is already swollen. A teammate brings a towel soaked in hot water and places it on her arm. Meanwhile, your partner arrives with the trauma kit.

2. What is the benefit of the towel soaked in hot water?

There is no benefit! An injury that is accompanied by swelling needs either a chemical cold pack or a towel soaked in cold water. Applying heat to a swollen, painful deformity will cause vasodilation and increase the swelling, whereas applying a cold pack to the injury site will promote local vasoconstriction, which will serve to minimize swelling as well as provide pain relief.

3. Based on the injury location, what bones might have sustained injury?

The distal aspect of the forearm involves the possibility of several injured bones. This could be the radius and/or ulna (usually both), as well as the carpals (wrist bones). You should also suspect possible injury to the hand itself.

You remove the hot, water-soaked towel from the patient's arm and thank the teammate for her help. As your partner applies manual stabilization of the patient's arm, you assess distal circulation by capillary refill and sensory and motor function, all of which are present and normal. At the same time, you count her pulse rate, which is 120 and strong. She continues to cry in pain, which verifies a patent airway with adequate breathing.

4. What have you accomplished through these actions?

Not only have you performed an initial assessment of the patient (noting her airway as she was screaming and assessing her radial pulse), but you have also tended to her injury at the same time. In many cases when the patient is conscious and alert, the initial assessment as well as injury management occurs simultaneously. It is important to note that this is not always the case. If this patient were unconscious, the injured arm would have been your lowest priority. A more in-depth assessment of airway, breathing, and circulation would have been indicated.

While your partner continues to provide manual stabilization of the injured arm, you place a padded board splint under her forearm. The area of deformity has caused a void under her distal forearm, so you apply roller gauze to fill the void for support of the injury. Finally, you secure the splint in place with roller gauze and apply a sling and swathe for added stabilization. After splinting the injury, you reassess distal circulation as well as motor and sensory function, all of which are present and normal. Her fingers were left exposed for this purpose.

5. With this type of injury, what joints need to be secured in order to prevent further injury and adequately stabilize the painful deformity?

With the injury site being the distal forearm, you will need to stabilize the wrist/hand as well as the elbow. Additionally, a sling and swathe should be applied to further protect and stabilize the injury. Remember, most patients with injuries to the upper extremities, especially the forearm, will prefer to hold their injured arm up against their chest. A sling and swathe will facilitate this.

6. How would you have managed the situation had distal circulation been inadequate or absent after splinting the injury?

First and foremost, you would have needed to evaluate how secure the splint was. Perhaps you applied it too tight, in which case simple loosening of the splint would have most likely fixed the problem. On the other hand, while splinting, you may have inadvertently manipulated the injured bones and caused compression of the radial artery. Had this been the case, gentle manipulation to restore distal circulation may have been required. Many EMS sys-

tems require medical direction prior to attempting this. It must be stressed that very gentle handling of an injury before, during, and after splinting is important; after all, the first rule of medicine is "First, do no harm."

After splinting the injury, you apply an icepack over the injury site. Meanwhile, your partner obtains a set of baseline vital signs. Blood pressure is 136/56, pulse is 112, and respirations are 20 and unlabored. After reporting the vital signs to you, your partner obtains a SAMPLE history, which reveals the following:

- S: pain and deformity to the right arm
- A: allergic to Motrin
- M: currently taking no medications
- P: appendectomy at the age of 11
- L: approximately 6 hours ago
- E: playing volleyball and fell while trying to return a volley

7. What components of the SAMPLE history, if any, are pertinent to this patient and her injury?

Her allergy to Motrin is a significant finding that is pertinent to this situation. Motrin (ibuprofen) is a nonsteroidal anti-inflammatory drug (NSAID) that is commonly prescribed to patients with various musculoskeletal injuries, especially those that are swelling. You must report this to the receiving facility so that the physician can choose another pain reliever for the patient. Additionally, Motrin is a trade name for ibuprofen. Other medications that contain ibuprofen include Advil and Tempra. It should be reported to the hospital that the patient is allergic to ibuprofen as opposed to Motrin. This will prevent the inadvertent prescribing of another ibuprofen-containing medication.

Your partner retrieves the ambulance stretcher and you begin to prepare the patient for transport. She asks to be transported to a hospital that is approximately 15 minutes away. You load the patient into the ambulance and begin transport. En route, the patient complains of increased pain due to the bumpy ride. You make the driver aware of the problem and she does her best to smooth the ride. You provide a bit more padding and change the icepack. You perform an ongoing assessment of the patient, which is unremarkable. Her vital signs remain stable. You notify the receiving facility and report the patient information as well as your estimated time of arrival. The patient is delivered to the emergency department in stable condition, with a report given to the charge nurse.

PATIENT OUTCOME/PATHOPHYSIOLOGY

The patient was diagnosed in the emergency department with a Colles' fracture to the right arm. There was no vascular or neurologic damage as a result of the injury. She was placed in a rigid, noncircumferential splint until the swelling subsided. She returned 24 hours later and was placed in a cast.

A Colles' fracture occurs when the distal aspect of the forearm (either the radius/ulna or the carpals) are fractured. Typically, this type of injury presents with a very distinct appearance that resembles that of a dinner fork or spoon; therefore, it is commonly referred to as a "dinner fork" or "silver fork" fracture. The patient with this type of fracture is at highest risk of vascular or nerve compromise. In small children (especially infants), this type of injury can actually lead to hypovolemia due to their relatively small blood volume as compared to adults.

EVALUATION

1. The most appropriate field term for a suspected fracture is:
   a. grossly deformed injury
   b. swelling, deformed injury
   c. swollen, painful deformity
   d. deformed, swollen fracture

2. Initial management for a patient with a musculoskeletal injury includes:
   a. assessing distal circulation and neurologic function
   b. manual stabilization above and below the injury site
   c. applying a temporary splint to prevent further injury
   d. manipulating the injury site in order to elicit crepitus

3. A Colles' fracture involves injury to all of the following bones EXCEPT:
   a. the radius
   b. the ulna
   c. the carpals
   d. the tarsals

4. The most appropriate splinting technique for a Colles' fracture is a:
   a. wrist sling and swathe
   b. short board splint
   c. a modified wrist sling
   d. a modified traction splint

5. Applying ice to a musculoskeletal injury promotes which of the following effects?
   a. vasodilation and increased swelling
   b. vasoconstriction and decreased swelling
   c. vasodilation and decreased swelling
   d. vasoconstriction and increased swelling

6. Vascular compromise from a Colles' fracture would be the result of compression of which of the following blood vessels?

   a. radial vein
   b. pedal artery
   c. radial artery
   d. brachial artery

7. The most distal point of circulation that should be assessed in the patient with an injury to the distal forearm is:

   a. the radial pulse
   b. capillary refill
   c. the ulnar pulse
   d. the palmar pulse

8. When splinting an injury to the forearm, you leave the fingers exposed for the purpose of:

   a. allowing blood flow to reach the fingers
   b. providing fresh air to the fingers to decrease pain
   c. assessing and monitoring distal circulation
   d. allowing the patient to be able to use the fingers

9. You are assessing a patient with an injury to the left mid-shaft humerus and note the absence of a distal pulse. You are 30 minutes away from the hospital. You should:

   a. provide constant traction with a splint to attempt to restore a pulse
   b. contact medical control and obtain permission to manipulate the injury
   c. splint the injury in the position found and transport promptly
   d. make repeated attempts to manipulate the injury in order to restore a pulse

10. A 37-year-old male who fell from his bed and landed on his shoulder complains of pain to the anterior aspect of his left shoulder. There was no loss of consciousness and there is no other injury. The patient has a patent airway with adequate breathing. Which of the following assessment modalities should be used?

    a. a rapid trauma assessment
    b. a detailed physical exam
    c. a head-to-toe examination
    d. a focused physical exam

33

My Aunt Has Fallen

Objectives

At the conclusion of this scenario, the participant will be able to:

1. Identify potential causes for geriatric falls.

2. List causes that predispose patients to hypothermia.

3. Identify mechanisms of body heat loss.

SCENARIO

You and your partner are washing the ambulance on a crisp fall morning when you are dispatched to a residence about 2 miles outside the city. The caller reports that she went to check on her elderly aunt and found her lying on the upstairs floor.

1. What are your thoughts concerning the dispatch information?

You reportedly have an elderly female who was found lying on the floor. Your first consideration should be what caused her to be on the floor. Did she suffer a syncopal (fainting) episode, seizure, cardiac dysrhythmia, hip fracture, or did she trip and fall? One of your priorities will be to identify the reason that she is on the floor. You should also be suspicious of trauma. No matter which of the above events may have precipitated the event there is the strong likelihood that she suffered injury if she fell. You should then focus on the length of time she has been on the floor. Elderly patients may suffer further injury due to their inability to get themselves from the floor. For example, they may be dehydrated if they have gone without water. They may have a low blood sugar if they have problems with glucose regulation. Finally, you must always consider the possibility of hypothermia in the geriatric population. Despite the ambient temperature of the room the body may lose a substantial amount of heat if it remains in contact with a cool surface such as the floor. Also, several medical conditions may predispose a patient to hypothermia. These include vascular insufficiency, diabetes, peripheral neuropathy, medication use, and alcohol use. The normal body temperature is 98.6°F. Shivering and difficulty speaking may occur when the temperature drops to 96°F and mental changes may occur when the temperature drops below 91°F.

2. What should you and your partner discuss while en route to the call?

You will need to decide which of you will perform which functions during the call. You will also need to discuss the method that you will use to extricate the patient from an upstairs area. In so doing you will save valuable time once you make patient contact.

You arrive on scene. You and your partner put on your body substance isolation (BSI) equipment, which includes your gloves and your eye protection, and grab your response bags and spinal-motion-restriction equipment. You approach the home, where you are met by the patient's niece who lets you into the home. You are cautious, as always, upon entering the residence. The niece informs you that she checks on her aunt at least once a day and that yesterday she was fine. She says, "Today when I knocked no one answered so I let myself in. She was lying on the floor and is not acting like herself." You are directed upstairs to a small bedroom where you see the patient lying in a lateral recumbent position on the floor. You estimate that the patient is about 80 years old and note that she is very thin. You direct your partner to provide manual cervical spine motion restriction as you introduce yourself and begin the initial assessment. You note that the patient is lying on a wooden floor, which is cool to the touch. You determine that the patient is conscious but confused as to her location. Her airway is open and patent. She is breathing shallow respirations at 16/minute. You note that her skin is very cool to the touch and that she has a weak, slow radial pulse. You also identify a "Medic Alert" bracelet, which states that she is an insulin-controlled diabetic.

3. What have you learned from this brief encounter?

Plenty. You have learned that the patient is confused and that this is not a normal state for her. You have identified that she is cool to the touch and has a slow heart rate with a weak pulse. You have also identified that she is an insulin-dependent diabetic. Items that are not clear include the length of time the patient has been on the floor and the reason that she got there. Assume that the patient may have been there since she was last visited by her niece.

4. What concerns have you identified?

Four major concerns have been identified. They are confusion, poor circulation, poor heat regulation, and a possible diabetic complication. You should identify that each of these alone is a serious event, but to have occurred simultaneously is a true emergency. You would be prudent to expedite transport to the hospital.

You initiate oxygen at 15 Lpm with a nonrebreather mask as you continue your assessment. You do note an abrasion with no active bleeding on the patient's scalp. Her pupils are round but sluggishly reactive. She denies head or neck pain. You identify no trauma to her thorax. Her breath sounds are clear and shallow bilaterally. Her abdomen is soft. You see evidence of urinary incontinence on her clothing. Assessment of her extremities is unremarkable except for some minor abrasions on her hands and severe redness in the areas in contact with the floor. Her distal extremities are very cool to the touch. Since she is lying on her side you are able to view her back and again note no injuries. You assess vital signs, which are: B/P 88/40, HR 52, RR 16, and an SpO_2 of 97 percent on oxygen. Her skin remains cool to the touch.

5. What should your next intervention be?

    Since trauma has been identified by the presence of abrasions you should begin to initiate spinal-motion-restriction devices. A cervical collar should be applied before she is log-rolled onto a long spine board.

    You apply an appropriately sized cervical collar and prepare to roll the patient onto a long spine board.

6. What should you do before placing the patient on the backboard?

    This patient is cool to the touch and may be hypothermic. You should place a well-insulated blanket between her and the backboard to prevent further heat loss. Patients lose body heat by one of five mechanisms. They are:

    - Conduction—the loss of heat by contact with a surface with a lower temperature than the body.
    - Convection—the loss of heat caused by air passing over the surface of the body carrying heat from the skin.
    - Radiation—the loss of body heat as it is given off to the surrounding environment like rays radiating from the sun.
    - Evaporation—occurs when a liquid medium comes into contact with the body. As the liquid evaporates into the surrounding air it takes body heat along with it.
    - Respiration—loss of heat caused by the warmth your body puts into the air utilized for ventilation. As you exhale air you lose heat that your body used to warm it.

    By placing a blanket between the patient and the backboard you will reduce the amount of heat that would be lost by conduction of her back with the wood or plastic.
    You remove the wet clothing that is soaked with urine. You then roll the victim onto the long spine board with a blanket placed between her skin and the backboard. You apply straps and a cervical immobilization device. You then cover her with blankets to reduce the risk of further heat loss and to provide passive rewarming. You are aware that since she is a diabetic and is confused, you should administer a dose of "instant-glucose."

7. Will you administer the instant-glucose? If so, how will you administer it?

    Since the victim is confused and you do suspect low blood sugar, instant-glucose is appropriate. However, presently the patient is confused and lying flat on her back secured to a long spine board. One recommended technique for administration of the glucose gel is to place some on a tongue blade and place it between the patient's cheek and gums. Unfortunately, this patient is supine and may potentially aspirate the gel if given while she is laying flat. One technique that might be considered is to transport the patient to the ambulance and secure her, with the spine board, and tilt the board to the side. This would reduce the likelihood of aspiration and deliver the needed glucose as well.

You gather information about the patient's SAMPLE history from her niece as you begin to move the patient downstairs to the awaiting stretcher. You find that the patient has no drug allergies and takes only NPH insulin, a blood pressure pill, and multivitamins every day. Her past medical history includes her insulin-dependent diabetes and hypertension. You have no idea when she last ate. It may have been as long as 24 hours ago. The patient cannot recall what caused her to fall to the floor.

You move the patient to the ambulance and tilt the spine board carefully to the side. You then begin to administer instant glucose gel utilizing a wooden tongue blade.

8. What should you monitor for?

   Airway maintenance. Since you are administering the glucose gel you should be immediately ready to remove the wooden blade if she becomes nauseated or can no longer swallow or control her own airway. You will also need to reassess her and her vital signs.

9. What might you do to assist in rewarming the patient?

   If you have an oxygen humidifier that can be heated, you should change your oxygen-delivery system to the warming device. This will assist you in preventing the heat loss caused by respiration.

During your 8-minute trip to the hospital you do identify that the patient has an improvement in mentation. Her assessment and vital signs remain unchanged en route. You deliver the patient to the hospital where you give a detailed report of your findings, suspicions, and interventions. You and your partner depart the emergency department and prepare your ambulance for the next call.

PATIENT OUTCOME/PATHOPHYSIOLOGY

You deliver the patient to the emergency department with a slight improvement in her mental state. In the ER they identified that the patient did indeed have a blood glucose of 48 mg%/dL with the normal ranging from 90–110 mg%/dL. She was given IV glucose. Her rectal body temperature was also found to be 87°F. She underwent rewarming with a "Bear Hugger" heating system and warm enemas. Her x-rays were all negative and no trauma, other than the abrasions, was noted. She was treated with rehydration and electrolyte replacement. She will be discharged in 5 days and will now reside with her niece and nephew.

1. Which of the following conditions may lead to a geriatric patient suffering a fall?

   a. seizure

   b. fracture of the hip

   c. syncope

   d. diabetic complication

   e. all of the above

2. Diabetes may predispose an elderly patient to which of the following conditions?

   a. gastric ulcer development

   b. urinary incontinence

   c. hypothermia

   d. kidney stone development

3. Convection is heat loss caused by:

   a. contact with an object that is cooler than the patient

   b. air passing over the surface of the body

   c. heat lost during exhalation

   d. heat lost through evaporation

4. Conduction is heat loss caused by:

   a. contact with an object that is cooler than the patient

   b. air passing over the surface of the body

   c. heat lost during exhalation

   d. heat lost through evaporation

5. Providing warm oxygen would decrease heat loss caused by which of the following mechanisms?

   a. conduction

   b. convection

   c. respiration

   d. radiation

6. Patients who present with mental confusion and have a diabetic history should be treated with:

   a. syrup of ipecac

   b. activated charcoal

   c. instant glucose

   d. Narcan®

7. Which of the following is of significant importance when caring for a patient who is suspected of being hypothermic?
   a. place the patient in warm water
   b. actively rub extremities to increase blood flow
   c. remove any wet clothing
   d. apply a heating pad directly to the skin

8. What is the most common fracture sustained by geriatric patients?
   a. humerus
   b. radius/ulna
   c. tibia/fibula
   d. hip

9. What is the normal body temperature?
   a. 90.1°F
   b. 95.2°F
   c. 96.8°F
   d. 98.6°F

10. With which of the following body temperatures would you expect to see alteration in mental function?
    a. 90.1°F
    b. 95.2°F
    c. 96.8°F
    d. 98.6°F

34

A FALL AT A
CONSTRUCTION SITE

Objectives

At the conclusion of this scenario, the participant will be able to:

1. Identify possible situations that could cause an unsafe scene.

2. Describe techniques utilized to assess trauma patients.

3. Discuss contraindications to traction splint application.

SCENARIO

Your ambulance has been dispatched to a new-house construction site for a reported fall. The caller stated that one of the men fell from a ladder while working on a ceiling. He is said to be awake and in a lot of pain.

1. What are your thoughts concerning this dispatch information?

   You are reassured by the report that the patient is awake at the time of the call. Your next concern should turn to that of your safety. New-home construction sites are often dangerous locations. Therefore, you will need to be very observant for your safety and that of your partner. Your next concern should be that of the fall. You will need to keep a high index of suspicion for spinal involvement with this type of injury. Be prepared to provide spinal motion restriction as necessary.

2. What equipment should you prepare to carry with you to the patient's side?

   You will obviously carry in your first-response bags, which should include the necessary items to deal with the airway. Trauma equipment may be necessary. You should always carry oxygen and delivery devices to every patient contact. Since this is a reported fall, you would also be prudent to carry items necessary to provide spinal motion restriction as well. And, as with all calls, you will need to get your personal protective equipment for body substance isolation (BSI). BSI equipment should include gloves and eye protection.

You arrive on scene and gather your equipment before entering the home. The home is about midway through its construction and there are many areas of concern with wires, conduit, loose lumber, and electrical equipment all around. There is a lot of other equipment lying on the concrete flooring. You are very careful as you make your way to the patient. You direct other workers to clear a path for the stretcher. You arrive in the living area of the home. There you see a 20-foot ladder lying on the floor and next to it is the patient. You identify that the patient is conscious and alert so you obtain informed consent to treat.

3. What information have you gathered from this brief encounter?

   You have determined that the patient is conscious and alert. You have also determined that the patient could have suffered a fall from as far up as 20 feet depending upon his location on the ladder. You also identified that the surface the worker fell upon is concrete. You know that this is one of the most "unforgiving" structures that you could land upon. As you are aware, falls of greater than 15 feet, or three times that of the height of the patient, are of great concern. This is a serious mechanism and one that may cause severe injury.

4. What will you do next?

   Your next concern should be that of suspected spinal injury. You should direct your partner, if available, to perform manual head- and neck-motion restriction. If your partner is not available then you should perform this function yourself.

   Your partner begins to hold manual stabilization of the cervical spine. You perform a quick survey of the ABCs. You again note that the patient is conscious and alert. His airway remains open/patent and his breathing is unlabored. You are able to palpate a strong radial pulse. You also identify no sources of external bleeding. You do see deformity to both the right thigh and right lower leg. You continue with your focused history and physical exam. You ask the patient what happened and where he is hurting. He tells you that he was on the very top of the ladder extending his body when the ladder began to tilt and fall. He tells you that he hurts in his lower back and his right leg.

5. What should your next question be?

   You should ask the patient which part of his body hit the ground and whether he lost consciousness. Determining which part of his body struck the concrete surface can help you determine which way the energy was transferred. For example, we know that when someone falls from a significant height and lands on their feet then the energy is transferred from their feet and ankles to the long bones of the leg. This energy then may travel to the lower back and on up the spine. Determining whether or not the patient had a loss of consciousness may help in identifying a head injury.

You explain to the patient that you are now going to assess him from head to toe. You find no apparent injury to the head. Pupils are equal, round, and reactive to light. There is no blood or fluid discharge from the ears or nose. He denies neck pain. You bare the chest and find no visual abnormalities. Bilateral breath sounds are clear to auscultation. Assessment of the abdomen finds it to be soft with no palpable masses. Deep palpation, however, notes referred pain to the lower back. The pelvis is stable with no deformities or crepitus. However, again the patient complains of pain to the lower back during palpation. You find a deformity to the right mid-shaft femur area with no open wounds. You also note a deformity to the distal right tibia and fibula above the ankle. The patient does have distal pulses, along with motor and sensory function to both lower extremities. Assessments of the upper extremities are unremarkable except for some minor abrasions on the right palm. Pulses and motor and sensory functions are all noted along with equal grip strength.

6. What are your suspicions based upon your physical exam? What are your concerns regarding femur fractures?

   You are obviously suspicious of fractures of both the right femur and right tibia/fibula areas. This is evident by pain and obvious palpable deformity at the injury site. Remember that femur fractures may cause a substantial amount of blood loss. Some experts believe that you could lose from 2–3 units of blood (500–750 ml) from a single fracture. In the event of a closed fracture you can't see the blood loss. You may occasionally see some evidence of blood loss at the site if bruising is evident. Appropriate splinting of any suspected long-bone fracture will reduce the amount of pain and bleeding that can occur at the site. It is also known to decrease the chance of nerve injury at or around the fracture site. You should also be suspicious of potential lower back injury including a spinal fracture. Patients with referred lower back pain from either deep abdominal palpation or palpation of the pelvis should always be suspected of having suffered a lower spine injury. You would be negligent if you did not continue to provide good spinal motion restriction to this patient. You have also identified a positive sign. This patient may have a lower back injury but he remains "neurologically intact." This means that he continues to have good sensory and motor function below the level of his injury.

7. What should you do next?

   Since you have finished a rapid trauma assessment you should apply a cervical collar and oxygen to this patient (if not done in the initial assessment). Your next efforts should then turn to splinting of the right leg and provision of spinal motion restriction.

   You place a cervical collar on the patient while your partner continues to provide manual motion restriction. You also apply oxygen at 15 Lpm with a nonrebreather mask. You must now decide how you will splint the right leg.

8. Will you utilize a traction splint to immobilize the right femur? Why or why not? If not, how will you motion restrict the right leg?

   You should not use a traction splint for this fracture. Remember that a traction splint actually applies "countertraction." In other words it utilizes the ankle (via the ankle hitch) and the pelvic (ischial) bar of the traction splint to pull countertraction. It actually pulls force from the ankle and up the length of the leg. This would be fine for an isolated mid-shaft fe-

mur fracture. But, in cases of femur fractures that are either close to the hip or knee or have injuries to the distal leg, the traction splint is contraindicated. This patient has a suspected right lower tibia/fibula injury; therefore you will not utilize a traction splint. A better choice in this situation would be to utilize either a commercial device like an air splint or "Frac-Pack" in conjunction with long board splints or long board splints alone. Remember the general rule that we must motion restrict not only the fracture site but also the mobile joints above and below the fracture. Therefore an air splint or "Frac-Pack" would not provide motion restriction of the hip. Long board splints must also be utilized.

You enlist the help of several of the construction workers to help apply a splint utilizing long board splints and triangular bandages. You reassess distal circulation and sensory/motor function distal to the fractures and find that they have not changed. You are now deciding how you will transfer the patient to the long spine board.

9. How will you transfer the patient to the long spine board?

Some systems only advocate the "log roll" technique for placing a patient on a long spine board. Other systems encourage the use of a "scoop stretcher" to literally scoop the patient and then place him on the long spine board. Utilize the technique authorized by your system or that of your medical director.

With the help of the construction workers and your partner you log roll the victim onto the long spine board. His torso and legs are secured to the device followed by the head. You then reassess his neurological function and find that it has remained unchanged. You transfer the patient to the stretcher and begin transport to the ambulance. Once there you evaluate the vital signs and perform your SAMPLE history. Vital signs are: B/P 132/84, HR 110, RR 18, and an SpO_2 reading of 100 percent on oxygen therapy. The patient denies any allergies and does not take any medications. His only past medical history is a tonsillectomy when he was a child. He ate breakfast about 4 hours ago.

You continuously reassess the patient during transport. You give a radio report to the trauma center awaiting the arrival of the patient. Following your 10-minute transport you deliver the patient and a report to the team. You again assess the presence of neurological function to ensure that nothing changed during your transport. You depart and prepare your ambulance for your next call.

PATIENT OUTCOME/PATHOPHYSIOLOGY

The patient was assessed in the trauma center. He was diagnosed with a compression fracture of L4 along with fractures of his right femur and right tibia and fibula. He underwent surgical repair of his leg fractures. His spine fracture was deemed as "stable," meaning that no surgical intervention was necessary. However, he was fitted with a "torso brace" to decrease pain and further injury. He was hospitalized for 10 days during which time he underwent physical and occupational therapy. He is expected to make a full recovery.

1. How much blood can be lost from a single femur fracture?

   a. 100 ml

   b. 250 ml

   c. 1,000 ml

   d. 2,500 ml

2. Traction splints may be used on:

   a. the femur only

   b. the femur, tibia, and fibula

   c. the femur, tibia, fibula, and humerus

   d. any long bone

3. Which of the following would be considered a serious fall for an average-sized adult?

   a. a fall of 5 feet

   b. a fall of any distance that occurs on a hard surface

   c. a 17-foot fall from a roof onto grass

   d. all of the above

4. What should always be done following splint application?

   a. reassess distal circulation

   b. pull subsequent manual traction

   c. apply a pressure dressing

   d. remove dressings over open wounds to observe for bone movement

5. Traction splints may help to reduce pain and bleeding at the fracture site.

   a. true

   b. false

6. Which of the following are principles to follow when immobilizing a fracture?

   a. apply traction to any long-bone fracture

   b. never realign fractures that are severely deformed

   c. always motion restrict the joint above and below the fracture site

   d. never use an air splint on closed fractures

7. Which of the following statements about long board spinal immobilization is true?
    a. The head is secured before the torso.
    b. The entire board can be turned to the side if the secured patient vomits.
    c. Patients with a complaint of neck pain but a mechanism of injury that is not considered "significant" will not require immobilization.
    d. All of the above.

8. What should you consider doing for a severely deformed extremity fracture that has no distal circulation?
    a. load-and-go
    b. attempt once to apply traction and realign the bone ends
    c. apply an ice pack
    d. none of the above

9. Which of the following traction splints can pull traction on bilateral femur fractures?
    a. Thomas half-ring
    b. Hare traction splint
    c. Sager traction splint
    d. Klepel traction splint

10. Traction splints may be utilized on tibia/fibula fractures.
    a. true
    b. false

35

MAN STRUCK BY A CAR

Objectives

At the conclusion of this scenario, the participant will be able to:

1. Identify tasks that must be performed at the scene of a traffic accident.

2. Discuss components of the trauma assessment.

3. Describe appropriate treatment of patients suffering from femur fractures.

SCENARIO

Your ambulance is returning from a call when a bystander stops you to tell you that a man was struck by a car just around the corner. He tells you that he is up one block and on the right.

1. What are your thoughts and actions regarding this information?

   Your first thought should always be safety. This type of dispatch is not unusual. However, you must immediately notify your dispatcher of the call. Your dispatcher is your source of safety in the event that you need help. Your dispatcher needs to know your location. The dispatcher will also be responsible for notifying law enforcement and fire/rescue if needed. There have been occurrences in the past where emergency personnel were directed into a violent situation, so be careful.

   You notify dispatch of the encounter giving them a report of the nature and location. You also request dispatch of law enforcement and fire/rescue personnel. You turn the corner on the reported street and witness an adult male lying in the street. About 10 feet from the patient you see a parked car with damage to the hood and a broken and indented windshield. The driver is standing next to the car talking on a cell phone.

2. What information have you gained by the scene observation? What should your first actions be?

You have identified that one person is injured. The driver of the car is well enough to stand and talk on a cell phone so no immediate injury to him is identified. You have also identified the person lying on the street as an adult. Due to the damage pattern of the car you are suspicious that he was struck somewhere between the thigh and abdominal flank region by the front of the car. You have also determined that some portion of his body then struck the windshield. Also, because the patient is lying on the street, you have determined that there was a second impact when he was thrown to the ground.

You first actions should be those that increase safety for you, your partner, and the patient(s). Park your ambulance in such a way that not only makes it accessible for medical supplies but also makes it an effective traffic deterrent. You also need to use cones, triangles, or flares to ensure that you don't become the next victim.

3. What equipment should you carry with you to the patient?

The first thing that you should put on is personal protective equipment. You should wear gloves and eye protection at a minimum. You would typically carry your trauma bag to the victim along with oxygen administration equipment, portable suction device, long spine board, cervical collars, cervical immobilization device, and some type of restraint system.

Upon exiting the ambulance you ask the victim next to the car if he is hurt. He replies that he is not hurt, and that he is on the phone with "911." You ask him not to leave as you and your partner approach the victim lying on the street.

4. What are your first actions when you make contact with this patient?

The two priorities are consent and management of the spine. If the patient is unconscious then consent would be implied and you may begin treatment. Remember, however, that any adult who is competent may refuse assessment and treatment. You must assume that with this mechanism that cervical spine injury is likely. Early in your patient contact manual stabilization of the cervical spine must be performed and continued until such time that the victim is completely secured to the long spine board with a cervical-motion-restriction device.

You make contact with the patient who is awake and moaning. You introduce yourself and receive informed consent to treat. You explain to the patient that he should not move. You direct your partner to begin manual stabilization of the head and neck by placing his hands on the head of the patient. The patient is supine on the ground. You begin your primary survey. You have already determined that the patient is conscious and alert. His airway is open and patent at present. His breathing is slightly fast but not labored. He does have a rapid radial pulse that is palpable. You quickly look the patient over from head to toe, you see some minor oozing of blood from the right side of his forehead and right cheek. You also see a deformity of his right femur. You see no external bleeding from his thigh.

5. What information have you gained from this visual assessment?

You have determined that the ABCs are adequate at present. You have also identified that there is some soft tissue injury to the face and forehead. You also are suspicious of a fracture of the victim's right leg. You have not identified any areas where immediate direct pressure should be applied to stop external bleeding.

Fire and police units have arrived on location. They have secured the scene and firefighters have split in teams to recheck the driver of the car and to offer assistance to you and your partner.

6. What actions would you direct the fire personnel to perform at this time?

   You should direct those that are seeing the driver of the car to assess and get a refusal form signed if authorized in your service. Those that are helping you should be instructed to prepare the backboard for placement and to get the traction-splinting device from your truck.

You ask the patient where he is hurting. He states that his right thigh and face are hurting. You perform your trauma assessment as you direct a firefighter to apply oxygen at 15 Lpm with a nonrebreather mask and another to obtain a set of vital signs. You begin by quickly reassessing your primary survey. Again, you find the LOC, airway, breathing, and circulation to have remained unchanged. You assess the airway, which is patent. You examine the neck. The patient denies neck pain or tenderness. The trachea is midline and you find no deformity of the cervical spine.

7. What should be done at this point?

   You should direct a firefighter to place an appropriately-sized cervical collar on the patient if he is trained to do so. Your partner will continue to hold manual cervical motion restriction even after it is placed.

You bare and assess the chest. Some minor abrasions are noted. The patient denies any pain or tenderness to palpation. Clear, bilateral breath sounds are noted. The abdomen is soft with no guarding or tenderness. Assessment of the pelvis reveals no priapism and no pain or deformity to palpation. Assessment of the lower extremities reveals an isolated injury to the right leg. It appears that the patient has a mid-shaft deformity of his femur. There are no open wounds. You also note that distal circulation is present and that the sensory and motor function of his peripheral nerves are intact.

8. Why is the location and appearance of a potential fracture of the femur important to assess?

   Femur fractures are very serious injuries. It is estimated that you can bleed as much as 1-2 liters of blood in surrounding tissues from a femur fracture, potentially more if it is an open fracture. It may lead to hemorrhagic shock. Also, fractures of the femur that are either open, very close to the hip, or very close to the knee should not be subjected to traction-splint application. They are best managed with long board splint placement. This fracture, closed and mid-shaft, is an excellent example of an injury requiring traction-splint application.

You find that the upper extremities are uninjured except for some minor abrasions. Your assessment of the head reveals that his pupils are equal and reactive. There is no abnormal blood or clear fluid discharge from the nose or ears.

9. What is your next priority?

Your next priority is to place the traction splint and begin performing spinal-motion-restriction procedures. Trauma is a condition that is not treated in the field or even the emergency department. It should be thought of as a condition that requires an operating room. Short scene times are crucial in trauma care. Perform your necessary actions but be organized and efficient in time utilization.

Vital signs were reported as: B/P 112/70, HR 116, RR 20, PERRL (Pupils Equal, Round, and React to Light), and an SpO$_2$ of 99 percent on oxygen. You and an assistant place the traction splint on the victim's right leg.

10.   What should you do immediately following traction-splint application?

    Reassess distal circulation and neuro status of the injured extremity. Traction-splint application may cause impairment of circulation to the distal extremity. This is often caused by ankle hitches that are too tight. If you have noted a complication then you may have to readjust the splint equipment.

As a team, you log roll the victim and assess his back. You see only some minor abrasion with no complaints of pain from the patient. You place the backboard under the patient and log roll him onto it. The patient is secured to a long board with straps and head immobilizer.

11.   What part of the assessment should be performed now?

    None. The patient is in a spinal-motion-restriction device, so begin transport. Do not waste any further time on-scene. The remainder of the assessment may be done en route.

You place the patient on the stretcher and then in the ambulance. You immediately begin transport to the city's trauma center, which is about 10 minutes away. You notify the hospital of a trauma alert with an ETA as you return to your assessment.

You perform a SAMPLE history, which is unremarkable. The event that led up to the incident was reportedly that the victim was talking on a cell phone and wasn't paying attention as he crossed the street. He didn't see the car coming as he stepped out in front of it. The car, he estimates, was going about 30 mph when it struck him on the right leg. He then rolled up onto the hood, striking his face on the windshield. As the car braked he was then thrown to the ground. He asks if anyone can get his cell phone from the driver of the car as he borrowed it to call "911."

You deliver the victim to the trauma center without any further incident. You give report to the trauma team before going to clean your ambulance. You wait around long enough to get your traction splint back—you know that if you didn't you would never see it again.

PATIENT OUTCOME/PATHOPHYSIOLOGY

The trauma team evaluated your patient. The CT scan of his brain was negative for any bleeding or swelling. All other exams revealed that he did in fact break his right femur along with his right xygomatic (cheek) bone. He was started on IV antibiotics and underwent a rod-insertion procedure in the operating room (OR) to stabilize his right femur. He was hospitalized for 9 days before discharge. Occupational and physical therapy was administered during his stay. His cell phone was never recovered.

1. What is your first priority at the scene of an automobile versus pedestrian accident?

    a. assessment of level of consciousness

    b. manual stabilization of the cervical spine

    c. assessment and management of the airway

    d. scene safety

2. How much blood may be lost from a femur fracture?

    a. 100 ml

    b. 250 ml

    c. 2,500 ml

    d. 1 liter

3. If a patient were found unconscious at the scene of an accident you would begin treating him under the auspices of which type of consent?

    a. informed

    b. unconscious

    c. implied

    d. good Samaritan

4. Femur fractures that are open and close to the knee should be treated with which type of splint?

    a. traction splint

    b. long board splint

    c. air splint

    d. M.A.S.T. pants

5. You should remain on-scene to perform a detailed assessment on every victim of trauma.

    a. true

    b. false

6. Priapism, a persistent penile erection, may indicate what type of injury?

    a. pelvic fracture

    b. vascular compromise

    c. testicular torsion

    d. spinal injury

7. If you are first at the scene of a traffic-related accident, one of your first priorities is:

    a. evidence collection
    b. gaining access to the victim
    c. scene security by appropriately detouring or stopping traffic
    d. parking your ambulance as close to the victim as possible

8. Blood or clear fluid drainage from the ears or nose of a trauma victim may indicate which of the following?

    a. severe infection
    b. brain swelling
    c. epidural hematoma
    d. basilar skull fracture

9. When opening the airway of a trauma victim you should utilize which of the following techniques?

    a. head tilt – chin lift
    b. neck hyperextension – chin lift
    c. modified jaw thrust
    d. none of the above

10. Patients who suffer from serious traumatic injuries are best cared for by which of the following facilities?

    a. the closest medical clinic
    b. the closest hospital
    c. regional trauma hospital
    d. any of the above

36

SHE FELL SOMETIME LAST NIGHT

Objectives

At the conclusion of this scenario, the participant will be able to:

1. Describe the assessment techniques for the geriatric patient.

2. List the signs and symptoms of a hip injury.

3. Describe how to manage the geriatric patient with a hip injury.

SCENARIO

At approximately 0540, you receive a call to a local nursing home where a 78-year-old woman has fallen. They are unsure if she sustained any injuries and would like EMS to evaluate her.

1. What are some concerns with trauma in the elderly?

   Unlike their younger counterparts, relatively minor trauma can result in significant injuries in the elderly. Through the natural process of aging, the bones become more brittle as a result of chronic calcium deficiencies. This makes them more prone to fracture from even the most minor trauma.

   Additionally, due to a loss of coordination, balance, and equilibrium, geriatric patients lose the ability to catch themselves as they fall. With this patient and all geriatric patients, you should be suspicious for a variety of injuries.

   You arrive on scene at 0550. A nursing attendant escorts you to the patient's room. You find the woman lying in the left lateral recumbent position next to her bed. You note that her bed is against the window. The woman is conscious, but not complaining of any pain. The nursing attendant advises you "She fell sometime last night." The staff did not want to move her in fear that they might worsen any injuries that she may have sustained.

2. Given the location in which you found the patient, what do you suspect may have happened? What would explain the patient's lack of any complaints of pain?

It is likely that this woman fell from her bed. Since her bed is against the window, she most likely rolled over, fell from the bed, and landed on her left side.

Remember, as we get older, our sensitivity to pain decreases. Serious injury can be present and the patient may not feel it. Do not assume that injury is absent in the elderly due to a lack of pain.

3. Due to the apparent mechanism of injury, what type of injuries should you suspect?

Given the mechanism, you should suspect injury to the entire left side of this patient's body, with the head potentially being the most serious. A careful assessment should always be performed on the elderly patient, even when there is no apparent or obvious injury.

You begin your initial assessment, which reveals that the patient is conscious and alert. Her airway is patent with adequate breathing. She has a palpable radial pulse at a rate of 64. Quickly scanning the body, you do not see any obvious bleeding. There are no signs of spine injury.

4. How would you manage this patient, based upon the results of the initial assessment?

Though you haven't discovered any life threats in the initial assessment, you should still maintain a high index of suspicion as you perform a focused exam of the patient. Since she landed on her left side, this would be the area to focus on. Oxygen therapy may be a consideration, should you discover any potentially serious injuries in your focused exam.

You carefully transfer the patient onto the scoop stretcher, after having placed a blanket on the scoop to avoid making the patient cold. With her now in the supine position, you check the back of her neck and find no injury or complaint of pain. You begin to secure the torso, legs, and head. You perform your focused exam of her entire left side. There is no obvious injury. As you are placing the straps over her lower extremities, you note that her left leg appears shorter than the right and is rotated laterally. The patient is still conscious and alert without complaints of pain.

5. Does this patient require spinal immobilization?

The mechanism of injury and assessment of the patient does not indicate spinal immobilization.

After the patient is moved onto the stretcher, your partner obtains a set of baseline vital signs. They are as follows:

- BP: 132/90
- Pulse: 64 and regular
- Respirations: 22 and unlabored

The SAMPLE history reveals no known medication allergies. She currently takes Vasotec (an antihypertensive medication) and a calcium supplement. Her past medical history is remarkable for a history of early Alzheimer's disease, peripheral vascular disease, and hypertension. Her last meal was approximately 10 hours ago and the events prior to the injury were that she was lying in bed.

6. With the shortening and lateral rotation of the left leg, what should you suspect and what management will you provide?

    Based upon this finding, you should suspect injury to the hip, be it a fracture, dislocation, or fracture-dislocation. Securing of the hip with straps and padding is the preferred method of treatment. Be alert! There is a potential for internal blood loss and shock with this type of injury so the patient should be monitored accordingly.

    After securing the patient to the scoop stretcher, you assess the affected extremity. You note that there is a weak pedal pulse present and the patient moves her toes as you touch the bottom of her foot with your pen.

    You place a pillow under the patient's head for comfort and she looks up at you and smiles. You apprise her of what is taking place and that you will be taking her to the hospital. The scoop stretcher is then placed on the ambulance stretcher; the security straps are placed and you begin to move the patient to the ambulance.

7. Why is constant communication with the elderly such an important aspect of patient care?

    Communication is an important aspect of patient care with all patients, regardless of age; however, in the elderly, they tend to frighten a lot easier due to the decreased ability to quickly synthesize what is happening to them in terms of your care. Additionally, the natural process of aging commonly produces visual and hearing impairments. This is a very frightening experience for patients as they have lost two of their most critical senses.

    Keeping the patient constantly aware of her surroundings as well as what you are doing is more appreciated by the patient than you will ever know. Patients need the reassurance of knowing that you are there to take care of them and that, in general, you care.

    The patient is transported to a nearby emergency department for evaluation. The trip is uneventful and the patient remains stable. You call your radio report in and arrive at the ED 5 minutes later. Care of the patient is transferred to the charge nurse.

PATIENT OUTCOME/PATHOPHYSIOLOGY

The patient's left hip and pelvis were x-rayed and the radiologist diagnosed a left femoral head (hip) fracture. The patient was admitted to the hospital and after a hip replacement and a stay of approximately 6 days was transferred back to a rehabilitation facility.

Hip fractures are one of the most common injuries unique to the geriatric population. The most common site of fracture is at the femoral head (greater trochanter) or at the neck of the femur. Due to the natural process of aging, chronic calcium deficiencies make the bones increasingly brittle and a process called osteoporosis occurs. For these reasons, the bones are more easily fractured, even as the result of minor trauma. Falls, due to a decrease in balance, equilibrium, and overall coordination, are the leading cause of hip injuries in the elderly. The most significant risk to the patient with hip fractures and/or dislocations is internal bleeding and shock.

EVALUATION

1. Which of the following is the most common cause of hip injuries in the elderly?
   a. falls
   b. motor-vehicle accidents
   c. spontaneous fractures
   d. elder abuse

2. Signs of a hip fracture include:
   a. lengthening and medial rotation of the leg
   b. shortening and medial rotation of the leg
   c. lengthening and lateral rotation of the leg
   d. shortening and lateral rotation of the leg

3. The most significant risk to a patient who has sustained a hip fracture is:
   a. extreme pain
   b. hypovolemia
   c. severe infection
   d. improper healing

4. An 80-year-old man has sustained a possible fracture to his right hip. He is conscious and alert and there are no immediate life-threatening findings in the initial assessment. The most appropriate next step in the care of this patient would be:
   a. a rapid trauma assessment
   b. obtaining baseline vital signs
   c. a focused physical examination
   d. providing full spinal immobilization

5. Common findings in the assessment of the elderly patient include:
   a. decreased sensitivity to pain
   b. an abnormally high blood pressure
   c. increased ability to comprehend
   d. increased visual acuity

6. When assessing an elderly patient with an isolated injury to the hip as the result of a fall, an important concern should be:

   a. how long ago the injury occurred
   b. the potential for other injuries
   c. what medications the patient is taking
   d. what care was provided prior to your arrival

7. The most common site of injury to the patient's hip is the:

   a. the lesser trochanter
   b. the mid-shaft femur
   c. the femoral neck
   d. the pelvic girdle

8. An effective means of moving a patient with a suspected injury to the hip is with the use of:

   a. a blanket drag
   b. a long spine board
   c. an orthopedic stretcher
   d. a full-body carry

9. Which of the following disease processes makes the elderly patient more prone to orthopedic injuries?

   a. coronary artery disease
   b. osteoporosis
   c. Alzheimer's disease
   d. peripheral vascular disease

10. You are transporting a 70-year-old man to the hospital for evaluation of a hip injury. He is conscious and alert with stable vital signs. En route, you should:

    a. perform an ongoing assessment every 5 minutes
    b. take a blood pressure and pulse every 5–10 minutes
    c. ensure that you maintain effective communication
    d. repeat the initial assessment every 20 minutes

37

I THINK I BROKE MY ANKLE

Objectives

At the conclusion of this scenario, the participant will be able to:

1. Describe the assessment of the patient with a musculoskeletal injury.

2. List the signs and symptoms of a musculoskeletal injury.

3. Define the techniques of management for musculoskeletal injuries.

SCENARIO

On a Sunday afternoon, your unit is dispatched to a local baseball park for a player with ankle pain. The time of call is 1450. You arrive at the scene at 1454. As you approach the patient, you notice that he is sitting next to second base and appears to be joking around with his teammates.

1. What have you gathered from your general impression of the patient?

   The patient joking with his teammates would certainly indicate an oriented and potentially stable patient. Remember, the general impression is a first impression of the patient. The patient's noncritical appearance does not rule out the fact that he is injured.

   After donning your gloves, you make contact with the patient, who is holding his left foot and ankle. He states that he was rounding second base when his foot slipped off of the bag and he twisted his ankle. He continues laughing with his friends and states, "But really, it hurts, and I think I broke my ankle." Your partner provides manual stabilization of the injured ankle, exposes the foot, and assesses distal circulation. The patient has a strong pedal pulse at a rate of approximately 90.

2. What are your initial assessment findings?

In patients that are obviously stable with an isolated injury, the initial assessment usually occurs simply by talking to the patient. The fact that he is oriented, talking, and laughing verifies a patent airway with adequate breathing. The fact that he has a palpable pedal pulse at a normal rate indicates adequate perfusion.

3. Based on the information provided by the patient, how would you describe the mechanism of injury?

From what the patient tells you, he has most likely sustained an inversion injury to the ankle. An inversion injury occurs when the ankle twists inward. The site of injury and pain with this type of injury is usually to the lateral aspect of the foot and ankle.

Determining that a focused physical exam of the ankle is indicated, you begin to assess the injury site. The patient complains of pain to the lateral aspect of his left foot. There is marked swelling and ecchymosis along the entire lateral aspect of his foot. You again assess distal circulation and find a strong pedal pulse as well as intact neurovascular status, as the patient is able to wiggle his toes. There is no other obvious injury noted to the left extremity.

4. What assessment findings are suggestive of a fracture?

Ecchymosis, swelling, and pain are all suggestive of a fracture; however, fractures are neither ruled out nor ruled in by the EMT. The presence of a fracture can only be diagnosed by x-ray. Since the EMT does not have this capability in the field, and because the swelling might cover any subtle deformity, fracture should be assumed and managed accordingly.

As your partner cradles the injured foot/ankle in a pillow from the ambulance, you obtain a set of baseline vital signs. His blood pressure is 116/70, pulse is 88, and respirations are 18 and unlabored. The SAMPLE history is unremarkable. Upon completing splinting of the injury, your partner advises you that distal circulation and sensory and motor function remain intact.

5. What is the advantage of a pillow splint over an air splint for a musculoskeletal injury that is swelling?

First of all, injuries that are actively swelling should not be splinted by materials that will provide circumferential inward pressure (e.g., air splint). This could result in compromise in circulation to the injury site. For this type of injury specifically, a pillow splint is ideal as it provides total support of the entire injury without restricting further swelling. In addition, ice can be applied, which results in local vasoconstriction and will limit the amount of swelling as well as help with the pain.

Your partner is obtaining the patient's information for the patient care form. You ask the patient if he wishes to be transported to the hospital via EMS. He states that he would rather contact his personal physician and have him meet him at his office since his physician has an "x-ray machine." He requests that you transport him there via ambulance.

6. Is this a reasonable request of the patient?

Possibly. EMTs should transport a patient to the health-care facility of their choice. This is not necessarily always a hospital. Many insurance companies prefer transport to their urgent care centers for injuries like this. The final caveat is that the patient doesn't always know best. In the case of an open fracture or more serious injuries (e.g., two fractures) hospital care is warranted. Of course you must follow your local protocols. Medical direction is also available to help with the decision.

7. How will you accommodate this patient's request?

If the physician can provide the care that the patient needs (x-ray, casting of the injury if needed), you should contact the patient's physician and transport to his office. Getting approval from medical direction and following local protocols is also important.

You place the patient on the stretcher and proceed to the ambulance. The patient's exit is met with a round of applause by the crowd. Your partner has since contacted the patient's physician, who said that he would be happy to see him. Your estimated transport time to the physician's office is 6 minutes.

8. What will your management of the patient consist of while en route to the physician's office?

With such a short transport time, as well as the stability of the patient, supportive care and monitoring of distal motor, sensory function, and circulation in the injury site would be the most appropriate management during transport. Remember, stable patients should have repeat assessments every 15 minutes. You are 6 minutes from the physician's office, so a repeat assessment would be limited.

Transport of the patient is uneventful. When you arrive at the physician's office, the patient's physician, who assumes care of the patient, meets you. The patient thanks you for your outstanding service. You give a report to the physician and return your unit back to service.

PATIENT OUTCOME/PATHOPHYSIOLOGY

The patient received an x-ray at the physician's office, which revealed no obvious fractures. He was diagnosed with a sprained ankle, given Motrin for the pain, and sent home.

Inversion injuries to the foot/ankle occur when the foot twists inward, resulting in injury to the lateral aspect of the ankle/foot. This mechanism can result in a variety of injuries ranging from a sprain to a fracture. Signs of a musculoskeletal injury include pain, swelling, ecchymosis (bruising), deformity (the most reliable sign of a fracture), and crepitus (grading sensation of broken bone ends rubbing together). Depending on the extent of the injury (bilateral femur fractures versus an isolated injury), significant internal bleeding as well as neurovascular compromise can occur. The patient in this case study was given Motrin for his injury. Motrin (ibuprofen) is a nonsteroidal anti-inflammatory (NSAID) medication that helps to reduce swelling as well as provide pain relief. The usual dose of Motrin is 400–800 mg every 6–8 hours.

1. The most reliable sign of a fracture is:

    a. pain
    b. swelling
    c. deformity
    d. ecchymosis

2. Initial management for a patient with a musculoskeletal injury includes:

    a. manual stabilization of the injury
    b. assessing distal circulation
    c. taking baseline vital signs
    d. immediate splinting of the injury

3. Splinting techniques of a musculoskeletal injury that is actively swelling include all of the following EXCEPT:

    a. a pillow splint
    b. long board splints
    c. an air splint
    d. sling and swathe

4. Motor, sensory, and circulatory function in an injured shoulder should be assessed at which site?

    a. brachial artery
    b. radial artery
    c. femoral artery
    d. subclavian artery

5. An inversion injury of the ankle occurs when:

    a. the ankle twists outward
    b. the ankle twists inward
    c. the ankle is hyperflexed
    d. the ankle is hyperextended

6. What type of medication is Motrin?

    a. antibiotic
    b. anti-inflammatory
    c. steroid medication
    d. cardiac medication

7. The most significant complication associated with a closed musculoskeletal injury includes:

a. extreme pain
b. severe infection
c. vascular compromise
d. external bleeding

8. Which of the following statements regarding musculoskeletal injuries is true?

a. Significant swelling can mask underlying deformity.
b. If deformity is present, fracture should be diagnosed by the EMT.
c. Distal neurovascular status need only be checked after splinting.
d. Crepitus should be elicited by manipulating the injury site.

9. After providing manual stabilization of a swollen, painful deformity, the EMT should next:

a. assess baseline vital signs
b. splint the injury site
c. assess distal circulation
d. expose the injury site

10. Which of the following musculoskeletal injuries poses the greatest threat to life?

a. scapular fractures
b. unilateral femur fractures
c. bilateral femur fractures
d. open tibia/fibula fractures

38

HE WAS HIT
IN THE HEAD

Objectives

At the conclusion of this scenario, the participant will be able to:

1. Describe the assessment of a patient with head trauma.

2. List the signs and symptoms of a patient with increased intracranial pressure.

3. Describe the management of a patient with head trauma and increased intracranial pressure.

SCENARIO

You get a call to a local park for an "unconscious male." It is a Saturday afternoon at approximately 1604. While you are en route to the scene, the dispatcher advises you that the patient is a 28-year-old male that was hit in the head with a baseball bat. Evidently, the caller hung up without providing any more information. The scene is approximately 2 minutes from your station.

1. How should you and your partner prepare to handle this call?

   When responding to any call for an unconscious patient, the vulnerability of the patient's airway should be of paramount concern. Additionally, since this patient evidently sustained head injury, protection of the c-spine (cervical spine) must be concurrent with airway management. With the limited information, it would not be a bad idea to have the AED ready; after all, you weren't given any information as to whether or not the patient was breathing or had a pulse.

2. Are there any special concerns that you have based upon the limited information provided to you?

Absolutely! You have no information as to the circumstances in which this patient was injured. Don't assume that it is a baseball accident just because the patient was hit with a bat and it happened in a park. This could have been an assault. Have the dispatcher attempt to recontact the caller to obtain more information. In addition, you must wait for the arrival of law enforcement prior to entering the scene.

You arrive at the scene at 1605, where you see a police officer kneeling down beside the patient. The police officer looks up at you and states, "He looks pretty bad." As you near the patient, you can hear the snoring of his respirations. Your partner immediately assumes control of the patient's c-spine and opens the airway with a jaw thrust, after which the patient's respirations are no longer snoring; however, he is breathing very deeply and rapidly. A bystander states that the patient was "hit in the head" with a baseball bat by accident.

3. What has your partner accomplished in his initial actions?

Your partner has corrected two critical problems with the patient in one maneuver: protection of the c-spine with manual in-line stabilization and opening the patient's airway with a jaw thrust. As you will recall, unconscious patients do not have control over their own airway; therefore, the tongue will relax and occlude the hypopharynx (the area of the trachea). Simply using the appropriate technique (jaw thrust) will bring the tongue forward, thereby establishing a patent airway. Due to the mechanism of injury (hit in the head with a baseball bat), c-spine injury should be assumed and the appropriate stabilization measures taken.

As your partner gains control of the patient's airway, you assess respirations, which are deep and rapid at a rate of 36. He has a palpable radial pulse at a rate of 56. Upon evaluating the patient for obvious bleeding, you note that there is a large hematoma with minimal bleeding to the right parietal region of the skull. No other obvious trauma is noted.

4. What are your priorities of management based upon your findings in the initial assessment?

This patient has inadequate breathing and needs immediate assisted ventilation with a bag-valve mask and 100 percent oxygen. When assessing the airway to determine the most appropriate treatment to render, you must note the rate, regularity, and quality of the patient's respirations as well as the patient's level of consciousness. In this particular patient, he is unconscious with deep, rapid breathing. To help keep his airway patent, an oropharyngeal airway must be placed as well. Remember, no airway, NO PATIENT!

You should make note of the hematoma to the patient's skull, as it will serve to increase your index of suspicion for significant head trauma. However, since there is no severe bleeding it can be managed later.

Based upon your findings in the initial assessment, you realize that a rapid trauma assessment and prompt transport are indicated. You quickly perform a rapid assessment and find that the injuries are isolated to the head, that being the hematoma, and now small amounts of a blood-tinged fluid draining from the nose. Upon repalpating the radial pulse, you note the rate to be 48. As the police officer runs to the ambulance to retrieve your stretcher, you take a quick blood pressure and find that it is 190/104. With assisted ventilation in progress, you place an extrication collar on the patient and prepare for full spinal-restriction precautions.

5. In the management of this patient's airway, why would a nasopharyngeal airway be contraindicated?

The use of a nasopharyngeal airway is contraindicated in patients with obvious nasal trauma and those with nasal fluid drainage (cerebrospinal fluid) secondary to trauma, which is a potential sign of skull fracture. Insertion of a nasopharyngeal airway in these patients may result in inadvertent placement of the airway into the cranium itself, causing significant brain damage.

After complete immobilization of the patient, you place him in the ambulance and request that the police officer, who is a certified first responder, accompany you to the hospital. Prior to departing the scene, you obtain another blood pressure reading, which is now 204/112. None of the bystanders were able to provide you with a SAMPLE history, as they do not know the patient. You repalpate the radial pulse and find that it is now 40. You advise your partner to proceed with red lights and siren to the nearest trauma center, which is approximately 13 miles away.

6. What is the significance of the patient's vital signs?

Hypertension and bradycardia (low pulse rate) in the head-injured patient is an ominous sign as it indicates significant swelling of the brain. In fact, the triad of hypertension, bradycardia, and hyper/hypoventilation are a classic finding in patients with increased intracranial pressure. This triad is called "Cushing's reflex."

7. Will your management change based on the vital signs?

Absolutely not! The most important management that you can render to a patient with significant head trauma is aggressive airway management with assisted ventilation and you are already doing that. Additionally, you must ensure full spinal protection and rapidly transport the patient to a trauma center.

As with all head-injured and unconscious patients, you must be alert for vomiting and provide suction as needed. Many patients with significant head trauma go into cardiac arrest, so have the AED nearby just in case.

While en route to the trauma center, you advise your partner to call ahead to the hospital, as you are too busy managing the patient. You ask the police officer to continue ventilations as you perform a detailed physical exam, which is unremarkable. Again, the injuries appear isolated to the head only. Continuing with your present management of the patient, you arrive at the hospital and take the patient into the emergency department where the trauma team greets you.

PATIENT OUTCOME/PATHOPHYSIOLOGY

In the emergency department, the patient was intubated to further protect his airway and after brief stabilization, he was rushed to the CT scan, which revealed a large epidural hematoma to the right side of his brain. After surgical repair, the patient stabilized and was discharged 3 weeks later to a rehabilitation facility with some permanent disability, including partial paralysis to his left side and slurred speech.

An epidural hematoma, which is an injury located between the dura mater and the cranium, results from injury to an artery (usually the middle meningeal artery). The middle meningeal artery runs anteriorly along the parietal regions of the brain on both sides. Direct trauma to this area, as with the patient in this case study, is a common cause of this type of injury. In addition to the injury itself, a major secondary complication is an increase in pressure within the cranium. Recall that the skull allows for no outward expansion and will only accommodate minimal amounts of swelling of the brain. This puts pressure on the vital areas of the brain, especially the brainstem, which controls breathing, heart rate, and blood pressure. Rapidly increasing intracranial pressure will cause hypertension, bradycardia in response to the hypertension, and altered breathing as a result of brainstem involvement. Mortality is high unless the signs and symptoms are recognized early and the patient is managed aggressively with rapid transport to a trauma center. If left unmanaged, intracranial pressure will become so severe that it will force the brain through the foramen magnum (the opening at the base of the skull), resulting in what is called "herniation syndrome." This is usually a terminal event.

EVALUATION

1. Which of the following is most indicative of significant head trauma?
   a. the presence of an external hematoma
   b. a prolonged loss of consciousness
   c. a temporary headache without nausea
   d. hypotension and tachycardia

2. A patient was struck in the head by a piece of flying debris at a construction site. He is found to be unconscious with shallow breathing. Airway management for this patient includes:
   a. a nonrebreather mask at 15 liters per minute
   b. an oropharyngeal airway with a nonrebreather mask
   c. a nasopharyngeal airway with assisted ventilations
   d. an oropharyngeal airway with assisted ventilations

3. Which of the following sets of vital signs are most indicative of increased intracranial pressure?
   a. BP 90/50, pulse 68, respirations 20
   b. BP 160/104, pulse 56, respirations 34
   c. BP 158/100, pulse 120, respirations 6
   d. BP 70/40, pulse 140, respirations 32

4. An epidural hematoma usually involves injury to which structure in the brain?
   a. the distal carotid artery
   b. the proximal cerebral vein
   c. the meningeal artery
   d. the meningeal vein

5. The most important management for the patient with significant head trauma is:

    a. spinal immobilization

    b. rapid transportation

    c. elevating the head of the backboard

    d. aggressive airway management

6. A patient with potentially significant head trauma is conscious with adequate breathing. Which of the following management modalities are appropriate?

    a. placement of a nasopharyngeal airway

    b. placement of an oropharyngeal airway

    c. a nonrebreather mask at 15 liters per minute

    d. a nasal cannula at 4–6 liters per minute

7. An adult patient with serious head injury is at high risk for:

    a. hypovolemic shock

    b. cardiac arrest

    c. immediate infection

    d. serious tachycardia

8. The brainstem controls which of the following functions?

    a. posture and equilibrium

    b. speech and understanding

    c. breathing and heart rate

    d. primarily vision

9. Management for a patient with isolated head injury includes all of the following EXCEPT:

    a. 100 percent oxygen by the appropriate device

    b. elevating the foot of the backboard

    c. elevating the head of the backboard

    d. monitoring for vomiting and suctioning

10. If severe intracranial pressure is not managed, the result could be:

    a. herniation syndrome

    b. hypovolemic shock

    c. massive infection

    d. skull fracture due to the pressure

39

MY BABY CAN'T BREATHE

Objectives

At the conclusion of this scenario, the participant will be able to:

1. Differentiate between respiratory distress and respiratory failure.
2. Discuss interventions that will be necessary to manage respiratory failure.
3. Identify causes of respiratory failure.

SCENARIO

Your unit has been dispatched to a private residence for an infant with difficulty breathing. The caller, who is the patient's mother, states that the baby is not breathing very well.

1. What are your thoughts concerning this dispatch information?

There are many causes of respiratory distress in infants. Some of the most common causes are infections such as croup, bronchiolitis, and pneumonia. Other causes include conditions such as reactive airway disease, as is the case in asthma, and viral illnesses such as respiratory syncicial virus (RSV). One common cause in young infants is rhinitis, otherwise known as a sinus infection. Remember that babies are "obligate" nasal breathers. This simply means that they predominantly breathe through their nose. If they get a stuffy nose then they do not automatically convert to mouth breathing as adults do. Instead they may develop respiratory distress.

Respiratory distress is caused when the body requires a higher level of oxygen than it is currently receiving. If the demand is met then the distress will decrease. This is much different than respiratory failure. Respiratory failure is more severe than distress and oftentimes is the end result of worsening distress. Respiratory failure occurs when the act of breathing no longer meets the body's demand for oxygen. If intervention doesn't occur, death will follow.

Respiratory distress is not always initiated by a respiratory condition. It may be the end results of other illnesses such as dehydration, hypovolemia, cardiac complications, and shock. Sepsis may also lead to respiratory distress.

You and your partner prepare while en route to the call. You decide which of you will perform which tasks during the run. You then prepare by putting on your BSI equipment, which includes gloves and eye protection. As you near the residence you begin to assess the scene for safety. You grab your response bags and pediatric kit before approaching the home. You are met at the door by the patient's father, who directs you to the living area where the patient is being held in his mother's arms. The mother reports that the child, who is 8 months old, has been ill most of the day. He has had a fever, which has been treated throughout the day with Pediaprofen. He has also not been taking his bottle very well. The mother noticed that about an hour ago he was breathing a little faster than usual and that he sounded stuffy.

2. What have you identified as concerns from this limited report?

    You have identified that the child has been ill all day and has progressively gotten worse. You are aware that fever may cause an infant to lose fluid and may cause dehydration. You are also aware that fever in conjunction with a decreased intake of fluid increases that likelihood. Nasal congestion or "stuffiness" may interfere with effective breathing.

You begin your focused history and physical exam. You ask the mother to lay the child on the sofa so that you may observe him. You open his baby blanket and begin your primary survey. You see that the child is awake but does not seem concerned with your presence. He is not very alert to his environment. His airway is open with some sounds of nasal congestion. His respiratory rate is 42/minute. He has palpable brachial pulses, which are rapid at 170/minute. His skin color is slightly pale in color. His capillary refill time is at 5 seconds. You do notice some blue discoloration of his nail beds.

3. What is your impression from your primary survey?

    This child is very ill. You have identified that he is not very alert to his surroundings. Eight-month-olds are generally comforted by and will continue to keep an eye on their mother or caregiver. This child is also displaying signs of respiratory distress. You have identified that he is tachypneic with an RR of 42. He also has audible sounds of distress with his congestion. Most concerning is the blue discoloration of his nail beds, which would indicate cyanosis. Remember that over 50 percent of his circulating hemoglobin (oxygen-carrying product of the blood) does not have oxygen bound to it in order to cause cyanosis. He also has a capillary refill time of 5 seconds. In a child with a normal body temperature you would expect this to be less than 2 seconds. This is an indication of poor peripheral perfusion.

4. What should your next intervention be?

    Two priorities exist. First you should attempt to clear the airway of the source of his congestion. This may be done by clearing the nostrils with a low amount of regulated suction or with a bulb syringe. Then oxygen should be administered with high flow. You should already have identified this patient as a load-and-go patient. Short scene times are prudent.

You direct your partner to clear the nasal passages with a bulb syringe and to initiate oxygen therapy at 10 Lpm with a nonrebreather mask. You also direct him to assess vital signs. You continue with your head-to-toe exam. Assessment of the head reveals that the skin color is pale with some cyanosis noted around the lips. Palpation of the head reveals no deformity and the anterior fontanel is flat. The breath sounds are shallow bilaterally and you again note a rapid breathing rate. The abdomen is soft. The child's diaper is dry and the mother reports that she has not had to change it all day. Assessment of the extremities reveals cyanosis of the nail beds. The skin feels cool distally. You gather the SAMPLE history, which reveals that the child has been treated for ear infections but the last was 6 weeks ago. No allergies or medications are noted. The child is reportedly up-to-date with all of his immunizations. The child has not taken the bottle very well today. Your partner reports the following vital signs: B/P 58/30, HR 174, RR 48, and an SpO_2 of 91 percent on oxygen.

5. What should you do now?

    Begin transport. You have identified that this child is seriously ill and would benefit from rapid transport. The services that you can provide this infant in the field are limited. He will need immediate care by a physician.

    You and your partner place the child in an infant seat, which attaches to your stretcher. You cover the child with a baby blanket to ensure a normal body temperature. You continue to provide oxygen at 10 Lpm with a nonrebreather mask. The mother states that she would like to ride with her child. The father says that he will follow in the car.

6. Do you let the mother accompany her child?

    Children are best consoled by a parent. Also remember that when you care for a child you are also providing care for his parent as well. You should remain very professional and not fear having a parent with you during the care of their child. A parent may also provide an extra pair of hands when needed. A general rule is that a parent or guardian should be allowed to remain with their loved one unless their presence hinders patient care. An example might be that a parent becomes unmanageable when they see CPR being performed on their child; in this case, it may be better to escort the child to hospital alone and have the parent follow.

    You transport the patient and his mother to your ambulance. You secure the stretcher and have the mother buckle in as well. You begin transport to the children's hospital, which is 12 minutes away. You give a quick report to the hospital as you depart the scene. You repeat your assessment. You now see that the child's eyes are closed and he is not arousable. His airway remains open and now he is breathing 20 times a minute. You see a seesaw breathing pattern with his chest and abdomen. You also see that he now has an increased amount of bluish discoloration to his face.

7. What has changed in the child's condition?

    You have noted that there has been an acute decrease in his level of consciousness. It is also evident that the child has moved beyond respiratory distress and is now in respiratory failure. A decreased respiratory rate may not always be a sign of improvement, as in this case. All other signs also report to a worsening of his condition. Supplemental oxygen via a facemask will no longer meet the needs of the body. You will need to intervene emergently with a bag-valve mask device to prevent respiratory arrest.

8. What interventions, if any, are necessary?

   Immediate assistance with ventilation is required. Begin bag-valve mask ventilations with 100 percent oxygen via a reservoir attached to your pediatric BVM.

   You immediately prepare to assist the child's ventilations. You prepare the infant bag-valve mask and reservoir device by connecting it to the oxygen flow meter. You also open up the kit, which has several sizes of masks.

9. What is an appropriate size mask to use when ventilating the infant?

   The infant mask should be clear so that you can see if the patient vomits during ventilation. The mask should also be large enough that it covers an area from the bridge of the nose to the tip of the chin as well. You should also be able to "seal" the mask to the face during ventilation efforts. Ensure that the mask does not put pressure upon the eyeballs. This may cause eye injury and also cause stimulation of nerves that may slow the heart.

   You immediately remove the oxygen mask from the baby. You place his head in a neutral sniffing position and attempt to ventilate him with the bag-valve mask. You are unable to generate a chest rise and fall. You then reposition the head and attempt to ventilate again but again with little chest rise and fall. You then decide to measure and place the appropriate oral pharyngeal airway in place. No gagging is noted. Following its insertion you again attempt to ventilate and you now see good chest rise and fall. You ask your partner to call the hospital and let them know of the change of condition. You continue to assist ventilations at a rate of 24/minute. You compress the bag only enough to see good chest rise and fall.

10. What is the problem with giving too large a breath during BVM ventilations?

    If you compress the BVM too deeply or too rapidly you will cause air to enter the stomach. This causes the development of an air bubble in the stomach. If the air accumulates in large volumes or too quickly in the stomach then the patient may vomit and potentially aspirate the vomitus into the lungs.

    You continue to assist ventilations. You check a pulse and see that the child continues to have a brachial pulse. His color also appears to be improving with your ventilations as evidenced by a reduction in cyanosis. You arrive at the hospital, where staff meets you at the ambulance and helps you unload. The child is moved inside and then to an ER stretcher. The physician then moves to the head and inserts a breathing tube into the patient. The child is then ventilated with the bag-valve mask attached to the breathing tube. You and your partner complete the transport form and then clean the unit for the next call.

PATIENT OUTCOME/PATHOPHYSIOLOGY

The child was delivered to the emergency department with manual bag-valve mask ventilations in progress. In the ER he was diagnosed as having acute respiratory failure in conjunction with severe dehydration. He had a breathing tube placed and was started on a mechanical ventilator. He had two IVs inserted and then received several boluses of fluid. Lab work revealed that he did have an infection in progress. Following a lumbar puncture he was started on IV antibiotics. He was admitted to the pediatric ICU where he stayed for several days. He was removed from the ventilator following his improvement. He was hospitalized for 10 days before being discharged home. He is expected to make a complete recovery.

EVALUATION

1. Respiratory distress occurs when the body:
   a. has a respiratory infection
   b. requires more oxygen than it is currently receiving
   c. has too high of an oxygen concentration
   d. none of the above

2. A condition in which the respiratory system can no longer meet the needs of the body is called:
   a. dyspnea
   b. respiratory distress
   c. respiratory failure
   d. tachypnea

3. Respiratory failure can be treated with supplemental oxygen.
   a. true
   b. false

4. Which of the following conditions could lead to respiratory distress?
   a. sepsis
   b. pneumonia
   c. respiratory syncicial virus
   d. all of the above

5. A bluish discoloration that occurs when too little oxygen is bound to hemoglobin is called:
   a. hypoxia
   b. dyspnea
   c. cyanosis
   d. purpura

6. An appropriate-sized ventilation mask should provide which of the following?
   a. cover the bridge of the nose
   b. cover the tip of the chin
   c. provide an adequate seal
   d. not apply any pressure to the eyes
   e. all of the above

7. Which of the following provides the highest level of oxygen for the patient?

   a. nasal cannula
   b. simple face mask
   c. bag-valve mask
   d. bag-valve mask with reservoir

8. A decreased respiratory rate in someone who has been in respiratory distress is always a sign of improvement.

   a. true
   b. false

9. Which of the following are acceptable ways to review the normal vital signs for pediatric patients?

   a. EMS field guide
   b. Broselow Pedi Tape
   c. printed charts kept in response kits
   d. all of the above

10. Which of the following are signs of respiratory distress in a pediatric patient?

    a. tachypnea
    b. accessory muscle use
    c. increased work of breathing
    d. cyanosis
    e. all of the above

40

CHILD WITH TROUBLE BREATHING

Objectives

At the conclusion of this scenario, the participant will be able to:

1. Discuss the difference between respiratory distress and failure.

2. Identify signs and symptoms of acute epiglottitis.

3. Discuss appropriate prehospital treatment of a patient with epiglottitis.

SCENARIO

Your ambulance is dispatched to a private residence for a pediatric patient. The caller states that her 5-year-old son suddenly began having difficulty breathing.

1. What are your thoughts regarding this dispatch information?

You will be caring for a reported pediatric patient with sudden onset of difficulty breathing. You begin to consider the possible causes of difficulty breathing in pediatric patients. Any time there is a report of sudden onset you should consider the possibility of an airway obstruction. These are generally caused by foreign bodies such as coins, toys, food, or any other item that can be placed in a child's mouth. You must also be aware that there are some medical causes for obstruction of the airway. Conditions such as croup, which is more common in children up to the age of 3, generally have a gradual onset with fever accompanying the constriction of the upper airways. It may present with a characteristic "barking seal" respiratory sound. Epiglottitis is another medical condition that can lead to airway compromise. Epiglottitis is a condition caused by an acute bacterial infection that causes significant swelling of the epiglottitis. It is common in children up to age 6 but can occur in older children and adults. This may lead to a partial airway obstruction, which can deteriorate to a complete airway obstruction. Other conditions that may cause sudden onset of difficulty breathing include conditions such as an acute allergic reaction or reactive airway diseases such as asthma.

2. What should you and your partner do while en route to this call?

You will need to discuss who will perform what functions during the call. This will expedite your scene time and make your efforts flow more smoothly. Also, you will need to coordinate efforts regarding the parent(s). Children often respond better to our assessment if a parent is involved. You can also reduce separation anxiety by including the parents in every aspect of the call. Parents will also be one of your best sources of information regarding the onset and duration of sickness. Following this discussion you will need to gather your BSI equipment, which should include gloves and eye protection at a minimum.

You arrive on scene. You grab your response bag and pediatric kit before approaching the home. You are very cautious about scene safety. After you knock on the door the patient's mother lets you in. She takes you into the child's room. There you find the boy sitting on the floor. His legs are spread and he is leaning forward on his arms, which are locked straight. You are able to see that he has his head down with his chin extended. He has saliva dripping from his mouth. He appears to be working hard to breath.

3. What are your thoughts and concerns based upon this limited visual assessment?

This is a severe emergency. Children who are in respiratory distress who assume a set position to assist their attempts at breathing are in serious condition. Children usually allow saliva to drool from their mouths when they have difficulty swallowing it. This would indicate that the child is possibly so exhausted that he cannot swallow; however, this probably isn't the case since he is able to remain in this sitting "tripod" position. Another potential reason for drooling would be that he has a partial obstruction of the airway. This obstruction could be caused by either a foreign body or by soft tissue swelling in the airway. This presentation of a tripod position, respiratory distress, and excessive salivation with drooling is typical of the condition epiglottitis. This is a very serious infection causing rapid swelling (within hours of onset) of the epiglottis. The swelling may become so severe that it completely obstructs the airway.

4. How will you approach this patient?

You will perform a limited assessment and make every effort not to scare the child. Any maneuver that would cause the patient to cry, panic, or scream could cause immediate swelling and closure of the airway. It would be best to assess this patient utilizing the mother's assistance. You will also avoid placing anything in the patient's mouth. Something as simple as asking him to open his mouth and say "ahhh" could cause an airway obstruction.

You have identified this emergency as a potential immediate life threat. You will perform a focused history and physical exam as you prepare to expedite transport.

5. Which part of the assessment will you perform first?

As always, you will begin with your primary survey by assessing the LOC, airway, breathing, and circulation of the child. Again, however, you will do this in a nonthreatening and nonfrightening manner.

You get down to the patient's level so that you are eye to eye with him. You calmly introduce yourself and tell him that you are here to help. You ask him to look at you for a moment and he faces you. He appears very apprehensive and scared. He immediately looks back toward the floor.

6. What information have you gained from the assessment so far?

You have gathered a significant amount of information. The fact that you asked the child to look at you and he complied indicates that he has adequate perfusion of the brain. Therefore you know that he must also be oxygenating, at least somewhat, and circulating that oxygen. You will now need to continue your assessment.

You assess his airway and determine that it is presently open although he has an increased work of breathing noted. You also touch his wrist and find that he does have a radial pulse and it is rapid and strong. You find his skin to be warm to the touch. You listen to his breath sounds, which appear clear but shallow in all lung fields.

7. What intervention would you like to perform?

Begin oxygen administration. If the child appears calm and cooperative then you may be able to provide oxygen via a mask. However, at the first sign of resistance to wearing a mask have the mother hold a device and direct it toward the child by blow-by method.

You ask your partner to prepare oxygen at 15 Lpm with a nonrebreather mask. You inform the child that you want him to wear the mask and begin to put it on. He immediately begins to appear more frightened and apprehensive. He even tries to tell you no.

8. What should you do now?

Remove the oxygen mask immediately. See if the child will allow the mother to direct oxygen toward the child. If he continues to resist then make no further effort to administer the oxygen. In such a case you would simply prepare to assist his breathing if he became unconscious or stopped breathing.

You immediately remove the oxygen mask and ask the mother to get next to the child to comfort him. The child is calmed almost immediately. You ask the mother to direct oxygen toward the child with the use of oxygen tubing. She complies and the child appears to tolerate this well.

9. What should you prepare to do now?

You should prepare for immediate transport. This is one of the most serious medical emergencies that exist in medicine. There is no further benefit that can be gained by remaining on-scene. You will need to be very orderly and calm as you direct the mother and child to the ambulance. It may be best to allow the mother to carry the child to the unit. You may then secure mother and child on the stretcher or allow the mother to remain seated and hold the child in her lap. The latter seems to work best. Be prepared, however, to immediately intervene if complete airway obstruction or respiratory failure occurs.

You explain to the mother the seriousness of the situation. You explain to her that she must remain very calm and that her help is needed to ensure that the child does not get worse. She appears calm and is willing to assist you. You ask her to carry the child and to continue to direct the oxygen towards his face. You will walk beside her and carry the oxygen tank.

During the brief walk to the ambulance you begin to gather components of your SAMPLE history. She reports to you that the child complained of his throat hurting a little about an hour before she called you. He felt like he might be running a fever so she gave him some children's Tylenol elixir. He then went to his room to play. She went to check on him and found him in the position you saw. He has no allergies to medications. He doesn't take any medicines routinely. His only past medical history was a couple of ear infections when he was much younger. He last ate about 3 hours ago but he didn't eat much.

You arrive at the ambulance where you allow the mother to sit in the "captain's chair" and hold the child in her lap. She continues to provide blow-by oxygen administration. You begin transport to women's and children's hospital, which is about 10 minutes away. You attempt to take vital signs but the child again becomes very apprehensive and resistant when you place the blood pressure cuff. You elect to not take a blood pressure but will cautiously take a count of the respiratory rate and heart rate instead. You find his HR is 130 and his RR is 26 and shallow.

10. Will you transport the patient with lights and sirens?

   No! This type of emergency transport may cause the child to become more frightened or apprehensive, leading to potential airway closure. Prompt but nonemergent transport would be better for this child.

11. What should you do en route to the hospital?

   Continue to provide care that is nonthreatening. You should also call the receiving hospital and give them a patient report, which should include your suspicion of epiglottitis.

You continue to provide oxygen by blow-by. The child's condition remains unchanged while en route. Upon arrival at the emergency department you allow the mother to carry the child inside. Because of your radio report the emergency department is awaiting your arrival. They have also called an anesthesiologist to be by the bedside. Once you enter the hospital the physician states that he agrees with your suspicion. With no further discussion they have the mother carry the child, with them, down the hall to the operating room. You and your partner complete your run form and prepare your ambulance for service. You depart and return to your station, ready for your next call.

PATIENT OUTCOME/PATHOPHYSIOLOGY

The child was seen in the emergency department and diagnosed with acute epiglottitis. He was immediately taken to the operating room where he was given an anesthetic gas while being held in his mother's arms. This allowed him to relax so that he could be laid on the OR table. The anesthesiologist was then able to utilize a lighted fiber-optic system to place a breathing tube through the swollen vocal cords. While he remained unconscious they initiated IV access and began to administer antibiotics to combat the bacterial infection.

He was admitted to the pediatric ICU, where he remained on the breathing machine for 36 hours. After the swelling decreased in his airway he was removed from the breathing machine. He was discharged home 5 days later and a full recovery is expected.

EVALUATION

1. Which of the following conditions presents with a "barking seal" cough and is more common in children 3 years or younger?
   a. epiglottitis
   b. croup
   c. asthma
   d. otitis media

2. Which of the following conditions is caused by a bacterial infection that causes swelling of the airways within hours of onset?
   a. epiglottitis
   b. croup
   c. asthma
   d. otitis media

3. Which of the following positions is typical in a child presenting with acute epiglottitis?
   a. lateral recumbent position
   b. prone position
   c. supine position
   d. tripod position

4. In a child suspected of suffering from epiglottitis it is imperative that you examine the throat for foreign bodies.
   a. true
   b. false

5. Epiglottitis is more common in children up to which age?
   a. 2
   b. 4
   c. 6
   d. 8

6. When approaching a patient who is a child you should:
   a. stand above the patient
   b. kneel below the patient and look up at them
   c. remain at eye level
   d. any of the above positions

7. When caring for a child who has suspected epiglottitis you should always place the child in a supine position so that you can monitor the airway.

    a. true
    b. false

8. Which of the following methods is an acceptable method of administering oxygen to a child who refuses to wear a face mask?

    a. force the child to wear a mask
    b. bag-valve mask ventilations
    c. blow-by oxygen administration
    d. none of the above

9. Which of the following terms describe a condition in which the respiratory system no longer meets the demand of the body?

    a. shortness of breath
    b. dyspnea
    c. respiratory distress
    d. respiratory failure

10. Which of the following is the best method to transport a patient with epiglottitis who does not have a complete airway obstruction?

    a. lights and sirens
    b. lights only
    c. no lights or sirens
    d. sirens only

41

HE BROKE HIS ARM AGAIN

Objectives

At the conclusion of this scenario, the participant will be able to:

1. Describe the unique assessment techniques for a child who is suspected of being abused.

2. List the signs that are indicative of and should increase suspicion for child abuse.

3. Describe the management of the child with suspected abuse, including legal issues.

SCENARIO

You are dispatched to a residence in an upper-class neighborhood for an "injured child." The child is reportedly conscious and alert. The time of call is 1545 and you have a response time of 8 minutes. Upon arrival, you recognize the residence as one that you have responded to three times in the past 2 months. The family consists of the mother, her boyfriend, and three children.

1. What are your thoughts, if any, as you are getting out of the ambulance?

   You should be suspicious right off the bat since you have made multiple responses to this house over a short span of time. Your concerns should center on the supervision that these children receive. Be objective, yet observant.

   The boyfriend answers the door. As you enter the house, you find 12-year-old Johnny sitting on the couch, holding his left arm against his chest. You ask Johnny what happened. He glances up at the boyfriend, who states, "He broke his arm again" when he fell off his bike. You note that the other two siblings, a 9-year-old girl and a 3-year-old boy, are running around playing as though nothing were happening. They do not even acknowledge your presence.

2. What is "different" about this situation as opposed to other calls?

First of all, a 12-year-old child is certainly old enough to tell you what happened himself. The fact that he looks to the boyfriend in response to your question suggests that he is reluctant, or perhaps even afraid to speak. Second, it is typical for siblings to be curious and to watch the EMTs at work. These children act as though this is "just another ambulance call to their house."

You begin your initial assessment of the child. His airway is patent with adequate breathing. He has palpable radial pulses at a rate of 100. The child is fully clothed and you do not see any evidence of obvious bleeding. Upon exposing the injured arm, you note deformity to the left forearm; however, the boyfriend tells you that the child's injury is to the upper arm and that the deformity to the forearm is from an "old injury." Your partner begins to obtain a set of baseline vital signs.

3. What might explain the still-deformed "old injury"?

Clearly this injury was never treated and therefore healed improperly. This is certainly not consistent with care that is adequate for a child, or anyone for that matter. You must continue to be extremely observant with the rest of the assessment of this child.

As your partner advises you of the child's vital signs, which are stable, the child's mother walks in the door and states, "Johnny, I told you not to climb that tree!" The boyfriend gets up and walks into the next room. With the boyfriend now absent from the room, you ask the mother her version of what happened. She goes on to tell you that the boyfriend called her at work and said that Johnny fell from a tree in the backyard. As your partner is splinting Johnny's arm, you advise the mother of what the boyfriend originally told you. She has a surprised look on her face.

4. At this point, what are your thoughts? Explain.

There are clearly conflicting stories here. You should find it extremely odd that the boyfriend walked out of the room as soon as the mother arrived and scolded Johnny for climbing the tree, which totally contradicted what he told you. At this point, if not already suspicious for abuse of this child by the boyfriend, you should be. Be extremely careful at this point; you do not want to make any accusations or implications of abuse. You have established the following facts that have increased your index of suspicion for child abuse:

- Reluctance of the child to speak
- An old, improperly healed injury
- Siblings that are disinterested in your presence
- Conflicting stories between the mother and her boyfriend

5. What should be your course of action based upon your thoughts and findings?

The key here is how you should act based upon your findings. Your thoughts should be kept to yourself for now. It is critical that in cases of suspected abuse, the EMT report and act upon factual information. Report only what you see, hear, smell, or are told.

You must make a very concerted effort to convince the mother to allow you to take the child to the hospital, for he is clearly in a dangerous environment. In explaining the need for ambulance transportation of her child, the mother must be told that the injury needs immediate attention and that the child needs to be evaluated for further injuries.

As you explain to the mother the need for ambulance transportation to the hospital, the boyfriend reappears and says, "That's OK, we'll take him." The mother and boyfriend begin to deliberate the issue. The mother wishes for her son to be transported via EMS; however, the boyfriend is adamant about transport via their own vehicle.

6. How should you handle this transportation dilemma?

This is an easy one. The mother is the legal guardian of the child and wishes her child to go with EMS, so EMS transport it is. The boyfriend has absolutely no say-so in the matter. As an EMT, you only need permission from one parent to transport a child to the hospital. You should inform the boyfriend that you must adhere to the mother's wishes and transport via ambulance. If the boyfriend becomes uncooperative, you should notify law enforcement at once. Remember, as suspicious as you may be that the boyfriend abused this child, make no accusations.

After packaging the child, you place him on the stretcher and load him into the ambulance. En route to the emergency department, you notify them of your estimated time of arrival as well as the patient report. The child is delivered to the emergency department in stable condition.

7. What should your verbal report in the emergency department include?

In addition to the information pertinent to the patient such as any changes since your radio report, you must, by law, report your suspicions of child abuse to the emergency department physician. Remember, this is a legally reportable case and failure to do so constitutes negligence on your part.

After transferring care to the emergency department staff, you and your partner return to the station and prepare for a lengthy patient care form. You realize that you will probably have to write an addendum to the original report to ensure that you include all pertinent information and findings.

PATIENT OUTCOME/PATHOPHYSIOLOGY

The emergency department physician diagnosed the child with a left, mid-shaft humeral fracture as well as an old fracture to the left radius/ulna with improper healing. In addition, the physician notified child protective services, who intervened and handled the case from that point forward.

Child abuse is an increasing problem in this country, with the number of children dying consistently on the rise. Child abuse occurs in all races, both sexes, and regardless of socioeconomic status. This case study presented a common scenario, in which a "live-in" mate was the abuser; however, parents and other caregivers (other relatives, babysitters) abuse children as well. The best weapon that the EMT has in suspecting child abuse is index of suspicion. The EMT must be very observant when managing an injured child, especially if the situation seems unusual. Common signs of child abuse include, but are not limited to, the following:

- Multiple bruises in various stages of healing
- Bruises/injuries in atypical areas for a child (chest, back, upper arms and legs, etc.)
- Old fractures or other injuries that improperly healed
- Conflicting stories among caregivers as to the mechanism of injury
- Injuries inconsistent with the developmental abilities of the child
- Reluctance of the child to speak
- Other siblings in the house who seem disinterested

When managing a case of suspected child abuse, the EMT must never make accusations or implications of abuse because if you are wrong, you just set yourself up for slander. Instead, the law requires that you report your suspicions (based upon fact) to the emergency department physician, who in turn has a legal obligation to notify child protective services.

EVALUATION

1. The abuser of children is most often:
   a. the father
   b. the mother
   c. a boyfriend or girlfriend
   d. anyone can be the abuser

2. Which of the following is NOT a consistent injury pattern for a 3-year-old?
   a. pulled a pot of boiling water from the stove
   b. wrecked a go-cart while racing with a friend
   c. fell and lacerated his chin on the corner of a step
   d. hand or fingers slammed in a car door

3. Which of the following statements best describes the EMT's legal responsibilities with regard to child abuse?
   a. The EMT must notify the police immediately upon suspicion of child abuse.
   b. The EMT has legal authority to remove the child from the house if abuse is suspected.
   c. The EMT must report his suspicions to the emergency department physician.
   d. If abuse is suspected, the EMT should question the caregiver as to his suspicions.

4. Which of the following injury locations would be least suggestive of child abuse?
   a. the chin
   b. the upper back
   c. the chest
   d. the upper arms

5. A child was injured while skateboarding. The mother wishes for EMS to transport the child to the hospital; however, the father states that he will take the child himself. How should the EMT handle this situation?
   a. allow the father to transport the child
   b. transport the child based on the mother's wishes
   c. call the police and have the father arrested
   d. tell the mother that the father has the final say-so

6. When writing a patient care form involving a case of suspected child abuse, the EMT should:
   a. write down his opinion of the case
   b. include nothing of his abuse suspicions
   c. document subjective findings of the case
   d. write down only factual findings

7. Child abuse is generally confined to what socioeconomic status?
   a. lower class
   b. middle class
   c. upper class
   d. status is not related to abuse

8. Upon arriving back at the EMS station after delivering a child suspected of being abused to the hospital, you realize that you forgot to include vital information on the patient care form. What should you do?
   a. write the information on the original
   b. write an addendum to the patient care form
   c. nothing, as you have left the copy with the hospital
   d. destroy the original form and write another one

9. The EMT's best weapon when managing a case of suspected child abuse is:
   a. index of suspicion
   b. what the child tells you
   c. what the caregiver tells you
   d. your opinion of the situation

10. The initial assessment of a child suspected of being abused should differ from that of a nonabused child in which of the following ways?
    a. there is no difference
    b. you should focus on the injury first
    c. you should question the caregiver first
    d. the vital signs are usually taken first

42

CHILD STRUCK BY A CAR

Objectives

At the conclusion of this scenario, the participant will be able to:

1. Describe the assessment techniques for a critically injured child.

2. List the signs and symptoms of hypovolemic shock in the child.

3. Describe the techniques of management for the child in traumatic shock.

SCENARIO

Your unit is dispatched to the scene of a motor-vehicle pedestrian accident involving a 5-year-old child. Police units are already on the scene and advise you as you are en route that the child is "bleeding severely." Your closest trauma center is 50 minutes away.

1. What type of injuries should you suspect with this child?

   Severe! A 5-year-old child has a total of 80 cc's per kilogram of blood in his body, so he can lose much less blood before going into shock than an adult. Based on the mechanism of injury, you should suspect trauma literally from head to toe. A common injury pattern is initial impact to the left side of the body. In a 5-year-old, the primary point of impact probably ranges from the pelvis to the lateral chest, with the secondary impact being to the right side of the head as the child is propelled away from the car. Bottom line, you must be prepared to handle a critically injured child.

2. Are there any other special considerations here?

   If ALS assistance is available, it should be requested. Since the closest trauma center capable of handling severe trauma is almost an hour away, air transport is a definite considera-

tion. It would be wise to notify dispatch and have a helicopter placed on stand-by. The "golden hour" applies just as much to children as it does to adults.

You arrive at the scene approximately 6 minutes after dispatch. You find the child, a 5-year-old male, approximately 15 feet in front of the car that struck him. He is lying on his right side and is moving around slightly, but not making any sound. Bystanders have placed a blanket on the child. You see no obvious blood. A bystander is consoling the woman who was driving the car that struck the child.

3. What have you determined from the general impression of this child?

   The child being found 15 feet from the vehicle suggests significant impact. Second, although a blanket is on the child that may be hiding external bleeding, the lack of obvious bleeding suggests internal injuries. A silent child is a bad sign. You would expect a 5-year-old child to be crying when injured. This does not appear to be good.

Seeing that you are dealing with a critically injured child, you have the police officer notify the dispatcher to request the response of an aeromedical unit to the scene. You direct your partner to take control of the child's head and maintain in-line neutral stabilization. After placing the child directly onto a backboard, you assess his airway. The child is responsive only to painful stimuli. His airway is patent and clear of foreign bodies with respirations shallow at 36. His heart rate is 150, palpable only at the carotid artery. You note that the child's skin is cool, clammy, and pale. Making a quick scan of the child's body, you see obvious deformity to the left mid-shaft femur, but no bleeding is noticed.

4. How should you manage this child initially, based on your findings thus far?

   An altered-mental status with rapid, shallow respirations requires assisted ventilation via bag-valve mask and 100 percent oxygen. Tachycardia, absent peripheral pulses, and diaphoresis signify severe shock. At this point, the origin of the shock is not as important as recognizing its signs and realizing the need for a rapid trauma assessment and aggressive management. It should be noted that a unilateral femur fracture in a child this age is capable of causing shock secondary to internal bleeding.

The police officer advises you that the helicopter has an estimated time of arrival of 12 minutes. You perform your rapid assessment of the child and note the following findings:

- No obvious head trauma; pupils dilated and sluggishly reactive.
- No trauma to the neck, trachea midline; jugular veins flat.
- Chest is unremarkable for injury; breath sounds clear and equal bilaterally.
- Abdomen is rigid and distended.
- Pelvis is unstable with crepitation noted.
- Deformity and swelling to the left mid-shaft femur; pedal pulses bilaterally absent.
- Multiple abrasions to the upper extremities, no radial pulses; capillary refill 4 seconds.

5. What findings in the rapid assessment confirm the presence of shock (hypoperfusion)?

There are multiple findings that confirm your suspicion of shock. They are as follows:

- Dilated, sluggishly reactive pupils: caused by cerebral hypoxia.
- Flat jugular veins: indicative of hypovolemia.
- Absent peripheral pulses and delayed capillary refill: both signs of shock (hypoperfusion).
  - Capillary refill is a reliable indicator of perfusion in children less than 6 years of age.

6. What is the potential origin of the shock in terms of injury location?

   There are several injuries that you have discovered that could explain the cause of the shock:

   1. Rigid, distended abdomen: intra-abdominal bleeding.
   2. Pelvic instability: significant internal bleeding can result from this.
   3. Deformity of the left femur: easily capable of producing shock in the child.

   After completing the rapid assessment of the child, you place an extrication collar on the child and fully immobilize him. Additionally, you place a blanket on the child. Due to the criticality of the child, you elect to secure the femur and pelvis with straps and blankets. Continuing assisted ventilations, you and your partner load the child into the ambulance and prepare for departure to the helicopter landing zone. Just prior to departing the scene, you obtain a set of baseline vital signs. You are unable to obtain a blood pressure. The radial pulse is still absent, with a palpable carotid pulse of 154.

7. What is the significance of the unobtainable blood pressure?

   First, you should recall that the blood pressure reading is not to be relied upon as an indicator of perfusion, especially in children (it is difficult to obtain). In shock, the body's compensatory mechanisms work to maintain the blood pressure. Even if you were able to obtain a blood pressure reading in this child, he has more reliable signs of shock (i.e., tachycardia, absent peripheral pulses, delayed capillary refill, diaphoresis, altered mental status, etc.). In this particular child, you will not be able to auscultate or palpate a blood pressure with absent radial pulses anyway. In managing this child, the PASG (pneumatic antishock garment) should not be considered.

   As you depart the scene, your partner gives a radio report to the in-bound aircraft, as you are busy managing the child in the back of the ambulance. You continue to assist the child's breathing and monitor him for signs of deterioration. With such a short response time to the landing zone and your dedication to the child's airway, you are unable to perform an ongoing exam of the patient. Upon arrival at the landing zone, a flight paramedic and nurse, who assume care of the child, meet you. Your total time from arrival at the scene to loading the patient onto the helicopter was 17 minutes.

PATIENT OUTCOME/PATHOPHYSIOLOGY

The flight crew intubated the child en route and intravenous fluids were started. Upon arrival at the trauma center, the child was diagnosed with profound shock secondary to a displaced left femur fracture, pelvic fracture, and a liver laceration. After brief stabilization in the emergency department, the child was rushed to surgery, where his liver laceration was repaired. He remained in the hospital for 13 days and was discharged to a rehabilitation facility for care of his femur and pelvic fractures.

Hypovolemia is the most common form of traumatic shock in both children and adults. Children are at a distinct disadvantage in that they have much less blood volume (80 ml/kg) and thus can lose relatively smaller amounts of blood than adults before going into shock. Additionally, injuries such as isolated femur fractures or even tibia/fibula and radius/ulna fractures can result in enough blood loss to lead to shock. This would not be typical in the adult. In smaller children and infants especially, head injury with intracranial bleeding can result in shock. This is due to their relatively large head in comparison to the adult; the infant or small child's head can accommodate large enough amounts of displaced blood to produce hypovolemia. Unlike adults, children have a tendency to compensate in shock for longer periods of time as compared to their adult counterparts. However, they give little to no warning prior to decompensating.

EVALUATION

1. The most common type of traumatic shock in both children and adults is:
   a. neurogenic
   b. hypovolemic
   c. anaphylactic
   d. septic

2. Management for a child in shock with adequate breathing includes which of the following?
   a. assisted ventilation with a bag-valve mask
   b. application of the pneumatic antishock garment
   c. rapid transportation to a pediatric trauma center
   d. supplemental oxygen via nasal cannula at 4 liters/min.

3. When a car strikes a child as he runs across the road, what aspect of the body is most likely to take the initial impact?
   a. the superior aspect
   b. the lateral aspect
   c. the posterior aspect
   d. the inferior aspect

4. A reliable indicator of perfusion in children under 6 years of age is:
   a. systolic blood pressure
   b. diastolic blood pressure
   c. presence of a pedal pulse
   d. capillary refill time

5. In examining a child's neck during the rapid trauma assessment, which of the following findings is suggestive of hypovolemia?

   a. distended jugular veins

   b. flat jugular veins

   c. bruising to the anterior neck

   d. a deviated trachea

6. Which abdominal organ, located in the upper-right quadrant, is most likely to bleed profusely when injured?

   a. the spleen

   b. the gallbladder

   c. the liver

   d. the stomach

7. As your partner assumes manual in-line stabilization of a traumatically injured child, you assess the child's airway. You find that the airway is patent and the respirations are rapid and shallow. The child is responsive to painful stimuli. You should:

   a. suction the airway immediately

   b. apply a pediatric nonrebreather mask

   c. provide ventilatory assistance

   d. assess for a carotid pulse

8. A late sign of shock in the pediatric patient includes:

   a. tachycardia

   b. restlessness

   c. hypotension

   d. delayed capillary refill

9. Which of the following injuries has a greater potential for producing shock in the child than the adult?

   a. head

   b. chest

   c. abdomen

   d. pelvis

10. Upon assessing a pediatric trauma patient that is not breathing, you assess for a radial pulse and find that it is absent. What should you do?

    a. begin chest compressions

    b. immediately transport

    c. assess for a carotid pulse

    d. elevate the child's legs

43

MY CHILD HAD
AN ACCIDENT

Objectives

At the conclusion of this scenario, the participant will be able to:

1. Discuss signs and symptoms of a closed head injury.

2. Describe the management techniques of patients suffering from closed head injuries.

3. Describe the effects of different types of closed head injuries.

SCENARIO

Your ambulance has been dispatched to a residential area where a child has suffered a bicycle accident. The caller, who is the patient's mother, states that her 10-year-old son was "jumping" his bicycle between two ramps when he struck his head on the asphalt.

1. What are your thoughts concerning this dispatch information?

You have been dispatched to a bicycle accident with possible head trauma. Your first thought is whether or not the child was wearing a helmet. Blunt-force head trauma is common in all age groups. The most common causes of head trauma are motor-vehicle collisions and falls. However, every age group has other causes. With children, play and recreational accidents are common. Head injuries are classified as either open or closed head trauma. Severe accidents may cause an open head injury if the force is sufficient enough to lacerate the scalp and cause concomitant fracture of the skull. The most frequent cause of open head trauma remains directed or self-inflicted violence with firearms. Closed head injuries are those that are sustained during blunt-force trauma. The significance of closed head injuries is based on either the direct trauma sustained by the brain such as contusion, bleeding, or coup-contra coup injures or swelling secondary to the injury itself. The cranial vault, which contains the brain, is a closed bowl, which allows very little room for swelling.

2. What should you and your partner do while en route to this call?

    You should discuss which of you will perform the different functions of the call. You will need to decide what equipment will be carried to the patient. You would be prudent to carry your first-response bag along with your pediatric kit. You will also need to carry your oxygen-delivery equipment and spinal-motion-restriction equipment with you as well. You will need to put on your BSI equipment, including gloves and eye protection.

    You arrive on scene near the home where you see a small group of children and their parents standing. As you drive closer you are able to see that the children had built a substantial "ramp" that is probably 4 feet high.

3. What have you learned from this brief scene assessment?

    You have identified a significant potential for mechanism of injury. Falls from bicycles that are operating on level ground is one thing; however, falling from a bicycle that may have been 4 feet or more off the ground adds substantial potential for injury. This may be a true emergency.

    You stop your unit and get your equipment before approaching the patient. You make it to his side, where his mother is holding him in her lap.

4. What concerns does this position cause?

    Your concern is that the child has been moved. If spinal injury did occur then further damage may have been done. You will need to be very thorough in your provision of spinal motion restriction. The mother may be able to help provide immediate motion restriction.

    You see that the child appears somewhat pale in color and has obviously vomited. He is trying to pull away from his mother and is verbally aggressive towards her. His words appear confused. You see that he is moving his arms and legs spontaneously in an attempt to move around.

5. What information have you gained from this visual assessment?

    You have identified that the airway is a concern. The child has obviously vomited and is therefore at risk of doing it again. You should protect him from potential aspiration by clearing his airway. You are also concerned about the obvious altered level of consciousness. Children, even those 10 years old, are usually consoled by the presence of a parent. This child appears confused. You have noted one positive item. The child is spontaneously moving his arms and legs in an attempt to move. At the present time his spinal nerves must be functioning.

    You ask the patient's mother what happened as you direct her to continue to hold him as still as possible. She reports that the children, without the parent's knowledge, had constructed this ramp. The other neighborhood children interject that he was really high in the air, trying to make his bike do a 360-degree turn in the air, when he fell off and landed on his head. He was not wearing a helmet. You begin your focused history and physical exam beginning with the primary survey. You have already noted that he is conscious but confused. His airway is open and there is no evidence of vomit remaining in his mouth or airway. He is breathing at 24 times per minute and it appears slightly shallow but non-labored. He has a radial pulse of 110/minute. You quickly scan him from head to toe and other than a contusion to his forehead you see no other significant trauma.

6. What should you do next for this child?

Begin oxygen administration at a high flow and prepare to provide spinal-motion-restriction application. You have identified that this patient is suffering from a possible closed head injury and will benefit from a short scene time.

You ask the child where he is hurting. He yells at you that his head is hurting. He also volunteers that what he sees is blurry. You direct your partner to initiate oxygen at 15 Lpm with a pediatric nonrebreather mask and then to apply an appropriately sized cervical collar.

7. What is your impression of his injury based upon your physical exam?

You are very concerned of a closed head injury. Some of the signs of a closed head injury include evidence of blunt-force trauma, nausea with or without vomiting, vision changes, headache, aggression, altered level of consciousness, combativeness, and unconsciousness. Initially the vital signs of patients will be completely normal. However, as brain swelling continues you may see an increase in respiratory rate. This is an attempt to reduce the brain swelling through hyperventilation. You will eventually see the heart rate begin to fall and blood pressure increase. These are ominous signs. If intervention does not occur quickly, death may ensue.
With this child you are concerned that two areas of his brain may have been affected. First, based upon the location of his contusion, you are suspicious of injury to the front part of his brain. This is consistent with his aggressive nature. The front part of the brain is a center that regulates emotions including aggression. Remember that the child who is uncooperative or combative is not in the right state of mind. These actions represent a continued worsening of his condition. You are also suspicious of an injury to the back of the brain at the posterior aspect. You are aware that the posterior brain is where vision function takes place. The child reports blurring of his vision. It is possible that the child impacted the front of his head causing a coup-contra coup injury to his brain. This simply means that on initial impact, direct injury to the brain occurred at that location but as the brain "sloshed" in its fluid home, it impacted the opposite side of the brain as well.

You perform a detailed head-to-toe survey. You find that the forehead contusion is the only site of trauma on the body. The child denies neck pain but you continue with the c-collar application. His pupils are equal but sluggish in reaction. He has clear bilateral breath sounds. His abdomen is soft with no complaints of pain. His extremities are clear of trauma and he has distal pulses along with sensory and motor function. His back is also clear of injury. You and your partner place the child on a long spine board and secure him in place with straps and a cervical immobilization device. You begin to move him to the stretcher in preparation for transport. During the move you inquire about his SAMPLE history from the mother. She reports to you that he has no medication allergies and takes no medications routinely. He also has no past medical history. He last ate pizza about 3 hours ago, which is consistent with what you saw on the sidewalk. The mother states that after the accident one of the children ran and got her. When she first got to him he was not awake but came around quickly. He gradually got more restless during the time it took the ambulance to arrive. He vomited the one time before EMS arrived.

8. What function should you perform next on-scene?

None! There is no benefit to be gained by remaining on-scene. The child has been placed in spinal-motion-restriction devices and is receiving oxygen therapy. Vital signs can be performed en route to the trauma center. Nothing would be gained by performing them on-scene. This patient requires emergent transport.

You place the patient in the back of the ambulance and sit the mother on the bench seat. Your partner begins the 8-minute trip to the trauma center. You perform a quick set of vital signs, which are: B/P 132/90, HR 118, RR 22, and an SpO_2 of 99 percent on oxygen. His level of consciousness remains unchanged. You give a quick radio report to the trauma center requesting that the pediatric specialist be notified. When you finish your report you see the child start to "dry heave."

9. What will you do for this?

You need to turn the board and the patient to the side. Even though he has vomited once he may still have food and contents in his stomach that he could bring up as well. Turn the patient to the side and prepare your suction device.

The child does not vomit. Once he stops dry heaving you return him to a supine position. The remainder of your transport goes well with no significant changes. You arrive at the hospital where you deliver the child to the trauma team. You give a detailed report to the staff and depart the ER. You prepare your truck for the next call. You feel good about your actions and your short scene time.

PATIENT OUTCOME/PATHOPHYSIOLOGY

The child was evaluated by the pediatric trauma team. The testing in the emergency department revealed that he did indeed suffer a closed head injury. The CT scan of his head revealed a contusion (bruising) on the frontal and posterior region of the brain. He was negative for any further trauma. He was admitted to the ICU for close observation. He remained confused for 2 more days but improved after that. He was hospitalized for 8 days before he was discharged home in normal condition. His parents did ban him from building bicycle ramps again. They also bought him a helmet, which he is required to wear during all cycling activities.

EVALUATION

1. Injuries that cause a laceration through the scalp and an underlying skull fracture are termed:
   a. closed head injury
   b. open head injury
   c. coup-contra coup injury
   d. cerebral edema

2. Aggressive behavior caused by a closed head injury usually involves which region of the brain?

   a. frontal lobe

   b. posterior lobe

   c. temporal lobe

   d. medulla oblongata

3. Visual disturbances caused by a closed head injury usually involve which region of the brain?

   a. frontal lobe

   b. posterior lobe

   c. temporal lobe

   d. medulla oblongata

4. Which of the following may be an early sign of a closed head injury?

   a. nausea

   b. headache

   c. vomiting

   d. all of the above

5. Which of the following is an ominous sign of a severe head injury?

   a. rapid respiratory rate

   b. equal pupils

   c. slow heart rate

   d. combativeness

6. Which of the following is the most important thing to manage when dealing with a patient suffering from a closed head injury?

   a. apply dressings to cuts

   b. apply ice packs to swollen areas

   c. manage the patient's airway

   d. take vital signs while on-scene

7. Patients who suffer from head trauma should be transported to a hospital that can perform a CT scan of the head.

   a. true

   b. false

8. Which of the following is the best method to administer oxygen to a patient who is breathing adequately and suffering from a closed head injury?

   a. nasal cannula

   b. simple face mask

   c. nonrebreather mask

   d. oral airway and BVM

9. Which of the following is the most effective method for decreasing the severity of closed head injuries in pediatric patients?

   a. classroom instruction on safety

   b. limit bicycle use to daytime hours

   c. training wheels for children less than 5 years of age

   d. helmet use

10. Which of the following signs may indicate a severe closed head injury?

    a. forehead laceration

    b. confusion

    c. unequal pupils

    d. headache

44

YOUNG CHILD FELL INTO THE POOL

Objectives

At the conclusion of this scenario, the participant will be able to:

1. Discuss risk factors that may lead to submersion injury.

2. Differentiate between drowning and near-drowning events.

3. Identify treatment priorities when dealing with pediatric submersion injuries.

SCENARIO

Your ambulance has been dispatched to the city pool for a reported pediatric drowning. Fire/rescue has also been dispatched for assistance. The caller reports that the child is about 9 years old.

1. What are your thoughts regarding this dispatch information?

Pediatric drowning remains one of the leading causes of pediatric deaths in the United States. There are several risk factors for submersion injuries. The age groups in the highest risk category include the very young (less than 5 years old) and those in their adolescent years (13–18). Boys have a higher mortality rate than do girls. Supervision seems to play an important role in the actual event. There is much less risk of drowning deaths in pools that provide lifeguard services.

Submersion injuries can happen in any fluid medium. Water injuries remain the leading cause. A very minimal amount of water is necessary. Small infants have been known to drown in as little as an inch of water. Swimming pools that are surrounded by fences will reduce the accessibility of small children. They are not, however, the only source of submersion injury. Any standing water may also lead to a drowning event. Five-gallon plastic

239

buckets have been identified as a leading culprit in the deaths of many toddlers who have the ability to get into the bucket but not get out.

This dispatch reports a drowning event in a public pool. We can only hope that they provide lifeguard services and that CPR was initiated in a timely manner. Also, be aware that spinal injury must be considered a possibility. Provide spinal motion restriction as necessary.

2. What should you and your partner do to prepare for this call?

You should decide who will perform what functions during the call. You will also need to take spinal-motion-restriction equipment with you to the patient's side. If your unit is equipped with an AED, and it is capable of assisting pediatric patients, then it too must be carried with you to the victim's side. Remember to wear BSI equipment throughout the call. Request that ALS start to the scene, if available, so as not to delay transport.

You arrive on scene just as fire/rescue is pulling up. You ask the firefighters to help your partner carry the equipment and the stretcher as you go directly to the patient with your first-response bag. You make your way to the pool area where you see a large group of people standing around someone lying on the cement. You make your way to the center of the group where you find a small child laying face down on the cement. Someone is straddling his back and pushing on his shoulder blade area. The helpful bystander tells you that he is trying to force the water out of his lungs.

3. What action would you perform now?

Have the bystander stop his actions. Hollywood has created many myths during its tenure, and copious amounts of water in the lungs is one of them. This maneuver has never proven to increase survival nor cause the patient to cough up large quantities of water. After you have stopped the bystander you should roll the patient onto his back with spinal precautions so you can begin your primary survey.

You stop the bystander from performing this action and log roll the patient onto his back. You immediately begin to assess the victim. You find that he is not responsive to any stimuli. You assess his airway, where you see evidence of vomitus in his oral cavity. You also note that the victim is not breathing.

4. What should you do next? Would you check a pulse first?

Your next action should be to clear the airway as you assign someone the task of stabilizing the cervical spine. You should then provide immediate ventilation. Only after the airway and breathing have been addressed does the circulatory status become important.

You direct a firefighter to manually motion restrict the cervical spine. You suction the patient's oral cavity of any visible vomitus. You then take your pediatric CPR shield and attempt to ventilate the child as your partner prepares the bag-valve mask device. You are able to generate chest rise and fall with each breath.

5. What should your next step be?

It is time to check for presence of a pulse. Now that you have opened the airway and have provided some form of breathing you should check for the presence of a carotid pulse. If there is no pulse then cardiac arrest exists and CPR with external chest compressions must be initiated.

You feel for a carotid pulse but you do not feel one. You begin to perform one-person pediatric CPR. You recall that you will utilize the palm of one hand that will be placed on the lower one-third of the sternum. You will compress to a depth of 1–1½ inches at a rate of 100/minute. Your ratio will be 5 compressions to 1 breath. You complete one round of CPR and then your partner is prepared to use the BVM to ventilate the patient. You now perform two-person CPR as you continue the 5/1 ratio. Your partner has also inserted an appropriately sized oral pharyngeal airway in place. If a pediatric AED is available it would be used immediately.

6. Should you be the one to continue chest compressions?

You have plenty of help available to you with the fire/rescue personnel. Effective scene management may dictate that you turn over this task to one of them while you continue to assess the patient for further injury or change in condition. There are still many tasks that must be completed. Consider utilizing your resources.

You turn over the chest compressions to one of the fire/rescue personnel. Your partner continues to provide ventilations with 100 percent oxygen via the BVM device. You stop those providing CPR and perform a pulse check but again no pulse is found. You ask them to resume CPR.

7. What should your next actions be?

You should provide spinal motion restriction and remove any wet clothing that remains on the child. Since trauma cannot be ruled out, you would be prudent to protect the spine from further injury. Removal of wet clothing is essential in pediatric care. Even in the middle of summer wet clothing can cause the patient to develop hypothermia. After you remove the wet clothing you should dry and rewarm the patient.

You apply a cervical collar to the child as you direct the remaining firefighters to prepare for long spine board application. You dry the child with a trauma dressing and cut off any wet clothing. You log roll the patient and following assessment of his back you place him on the long spine board, where you secure him with straps and a cervical immobilization device. You also apply blankets. You stop CPR again for another pulse check but none is found. You resume CPR.

You move the patient to the stretcher and begin transportation to the ambulance. You have been very efficient as evidenced by your scene time of less than 5 minutes. Once in the unit you secure the stretcher and prepare for the transport to the hospital, which is only 5 minutes away. You elect to keep a firefighter and your partner with you in the back of the rig. You ask another firefighter to drive the ambulance.

You have just initiated transport when you notice that the patient begins to vomit.

8. What should you do for his vomiting?

Immediately turn the patient onto his side utilizing the long spine board. This will decrease the likelihood of aspiration. You should also utilize a Yankauer suction device connected to wall suction. Reassess the airway and resume ventilations.

You turn the backboard to the side and clear the patient's airway. You also suction the mouth. Once clear, you reassess the patient and find that he has no spontaneous respirations and no pulse. CPR is resumed.

You continue CPR for 1 minute and reassess the patient. This time you find that the patient does have a palpable carotid pulse at 90/minute but is not breathing.

9. What will you do for this?

You will stop the chest compressions but continue the ventilatory assistance. You should breathe for the patient about 1 breath every 3 seconds to achieve a respiratory rate of 20. Continue to monitor the patient for a change including the potential secondary loss of pulses.

You stop chest compressions and continue to ventilate the patient at a rate of 20/minute. You arrive at the hospital before you have time to check blood pressure. You deliver the patient to the pediatric emergency room. There you give a detailed report of your findings and your interventions. The staff congratulates you and your team on the return of a pulse. You leave the ER and clean your truck. You then take the firefighters back to their station and thank them for their assistance.

PATIENT OUTCOME/PATHOPHYSIOLOGY

You delivered the child to the ER with a pulse but with no spontaneous respirations. You continued to ventilate him at a rate of 20/minute. In the ER he had a breathing tube placed and was started on a mechanical ventilator. IVs were initiated and he did receive medications to improve his blood pressure. He was admitted to the pediatric ICU where he remained critical during the night. The following day he took a turn for the worse. Despite numerous medications being administered he eventually lost pulses and was unable to be resuscitated. He was pronounced dead.

EVALUATION

1. Which of the following statistics regarding pediatric drowning is true?
    a. common in children less than 5 years old
    b. high incidence in children 13–18 years old
    c. higher incidence in males
    d. all of the above

2. Children can drown in as little as 1 inch of water.

    a. true
    b. false

3. You should suspect cervical spine injury in any unwitnessed drowning.

    a. true
    b. false

4. Which of the following items has caused an unusually high number of drownings in toddlers?

   a. dog bowls

   b. 5-gallon buckets

   c. hubcaps

   d. all of the above

5. When caring for a drowning victim which of the following will help reduce the risk of hypothermia?

   a. wearing two pairs of gloves

   b. turning on the lights in the back of the truck

   c. removing any wet clothing

   d. using a plastic backboard

6. While providing rescue breathing for a patient, he loses his carotid pulse. You should:

   a. increase your respiratory rate

   b. begin chest compressions

   c. perform the Heimlich maneuver

   d. none of the above

7. Where do we check for a pulse on an infant drowning victim?

   a. radial artery

   b. femoral artery

   c. brachial artery

   d. carotid artery

8. Where do we check for a pulse on a child drowning victim?

   a. radial artery

   b. femoral artery

   c. brachial artery

   d. carotid artery

9. Which of the following is the correct compression rate for a child drowning victim?

   a. 60/minute

   b. 80/minute

   c. 100/minute

   d. 120/minute

10. Overdistention of the stomach during bag-valve mask ventilation may cause the patient to vomit.

    a. true

    b. false

Appendix

Answers to Chapter Review Questions

Chapter 1: My Mother Is Gone
1. b
2. c
3. c
4. d
5. c
6. b
7. d
8. b
9. a
10. c

Chapter 2: She Is Having a Seizure
1. d
2. b
3. a
4. c
5. b
6. c
7. c
8. d
9. c
10. b

Chapter 3: Uh Oh!
1. c
2. d
3. c
4. d
5. a
6. a
7. c
8. b
9. c
10. c

Chapter 4: I Can't Breathe
1. d
2. c
3. c
4. c
5. b
6. c
7. b
8. c
9. a
10. b

Chapter 5: Difficulty Breathing

1. d
2. a
3. b
4. d
5. d
6. c
7. b
8. a
9. c
10. c

Chapter 6: It Is Hard to Breathe

1. c
2. b
3. a
4. d
5. c
6. b
7. d
8. c
9. a
10. c

Chapter 7: Unconscious Male

1. b
2. c
3. d
4. c
5. c
6. c
7. b
8. c
9. b
10. c

Chapter 8: I Think He Is Dead

1. b
2. c
3. a
4. b
5. a
6. b
7. c
8. a
9. c
10. a

Chapter 9: My Heart Is Skipping Beats

1. d
2. c
3. c
4. b
5. b
6. c
7. b
8. a
9. d
10. d

Chapter 10: I Have Pain in My Chest

1. d
2. c
3. b
4. d
5. b
6. c
7. d
8. b
9. a
10. c

Chapter 11: Possible Stroke

1. c
2. a
3. d
4. c
5. b
6. a
7. b
8. c
9. d
10. a

Chapter 12: Man Down

1. c
2. b
3. d
4. c
5. c
6. c
7. c
8. b
9. c
10. b

Chapter 13: My Son Had a Convulsion

1. c
2. b
3. c
4. d
5. c
6. b
7. c
8. a
9. b
10. c

Chapter 14: My Husband Is Acting Bizarrely

1. b
2. a
3. c
4. b
5. c
6. b
7. c
8. d
9. c
10. d

Chapter 15: I Am So Tired

1. e
2. b
3. d
4. c
5. c
6. c
7. a
8. a
9. d
10. c

Chapter 16: Unconscious Female

1. c
2. d
3. c
4. c
5. b
6. c
7. b
8. a
9. c
10. c

Chapter 17: My Daughter Ate My Meds

1. c
2. a
3. c
4. d
5. d
6. c
7. b
8. e
9. b
10. b

Chapter 18: I Think We Have the Flu

1. d
2. b
3. c
4. d
5. c
6. c
7. c
8. b
9. c
10. b

Chapter 19: Dizzy and Weak

1. b
2. c
3. c
4. a
5. b
6. d
7. b
8. c
9. b
10. c

Chapter 20: Feeling Weak at a Nursing Home

1. c
2. b
3. d
4. b
5. a
6. a
7. d
8. d
9. b
10. b

Chapter 21: I Am Having Problems Swallowing

1. d
2. b
3. d
4. b
5. d
6. e
7. b
8. d
9. d
10. a

Chapter 22: My Husband Was Stung by a Bee

1. c
2. d
3. a
4. b
5. b
6. b
7. c
8. c
9. c
10. b

Chapter 23: Attempted Suicide at the Jail

1. c
2. d
3. b
4. c
5. b
6. c
7. d
8. c
9. b
10. d

Chapter 24: My Stomach Hurts

1. c
2. b
3. c
4. b
5. e
6. a
7. b
8. b
9. d
10. c

Chapter 25: I'm Having a Baby

1. d
2. b
3. d
4. d
5. d
6. a
7. b
8. c
9. b
10. a

Chapter 26: Pregnant and Bleeding

1. a
2. d
3. d
4. d
5. c
6. b
7. b
8. b
9. b
10. c

Chapter 27: I Am about to Have This Baby

1. c
2. d
3. b
4. b
5. c
6. b
7. c
8. a
9. d
10. c

Chapter 28: Amputation

1. b
2. c
3. c
4. d
5. a
6. a
7. b
8. d
9. b
10. a

Chapter 29: I Cut My Hand
1. b
2. c
3. d
4. b
5. a
6. a
7. c
8. c
9. b
10. c

Chapter 30: I've Burned Myself
1. a
2. c
3. b
4. c
5. c
6. d
~ 7. b
8. a
9. d
10. d

Chapter 31: I've Cut My Arm with a Saw
1. b
2. c
3. d
4. c
5. a
6. d
7. c
8. a
9. d
10. a

Chapter 32: My Arm Is Broken
1. c
2. b
3. d
4. b
5. b
6. c
7. b
8. c
9. b
10. d

Chapter 33: My Aunt Has Fallen
1. e
2. c
3. b
4. a
5. c
6. c
7. c
8. d
9. d
10. a

Chapter 34: A Fall at a Construction Site
1. c
2. a
3. c
4. a
5. a
6. c
7. b
8. b
9. c
10. b

Chapter 35: Man Struck by a Car

1. d
2. d
3. c
4. b
5. b
6. d
7. c
8. d
9. c
10. c

Chapter 36: She Fell Sometime Last Night

1. a
2. d
3. b
4. c
5. a
6. b
7. c
8. c
9. b
10. c

Chapter 37: I Think I Broke My Ankle

1. c
2. a
3. c
4. b
5. b
6. b
7. c
8. a
9. c
10. c

Chapter 38: He Was Hit in the Head

1. b
2. d
3. b
4. c
5. d
6. c
7. b
8. c
9. b
10. a

Chapter 39: My Baby Can't Breathe

1. b
2. c
3. b
4. d
5. c
6. e
7. d
8. b
9. d
10. e

Chapter 40: Child with Trouble Breathing

1. b
2. a
3. d
4. b
5. c
6. b
7. b
8. c
9. d
10. c

Chapter 41: He Broke His Arm Again

1. d
2. b
3. c
4. a
5. b
6. d
7. d
8. b
9. a
10. a

Chapter 42: Child Struck by a Car

1. b
2. c
3. b
4. d
5. b
6. c
7. c
8. c
9. a
10. c

Chapter 43: My Child Had an Accident

1. b
2. a
3. b
4. d
5. c
6. c
7. a
8. c
9. d
10. c

Chapter 44: Young Child Fell into the Pool

1. d
2. a
3. a
4. b
5. c
6. b
7. c
8. d
9. c
10. a

INDEX

Violence, potential, 27, 121, 122
Vision, blurred, 235
Vomiting
  and carbon monoxide
      poisoning, 93–94
  inducing, 89
  in pediatric patients, 234–35,
     236, 241–42

  preventing aspiration by
     patient, 78

W
Warfarin, 170
Water breaking, before
  childbirth, 132–33

Weakness
  geriatric patients, 103–6
  heat exhaustion, 98–101
Wet clothing, and
    hypothermia, 241
Wheezing, 21, 23